The Complete MI Response Library

500+ Ready-to-Use Motivational Interviewing Scripts for Every Counseling Situation

Jane W. Harlow

ISBN: 978-1-7637425-9-8

Table of Contents

Preface

After three decades of practicing and teaching Motivational Interviewing, I've heard the same question from thousands of counselors, therapists, and social workers: "What exactly do I say when my client does X?" This question arises in supervision sessions, training workshops, and late-night conversations between colleagues who genuinely want to help their clients but feel unprepared for the complexity of real therapeutic conversations.

The gap between MI theory and practice has persisted since Miller and Rollnick first introduced this approach. While we understand the principles—express empathy, develop discrepancy, roll with resistance, support self-efficacy—translating these concepts into actual words in the heat of a difficult session remains challenging. Too many practitioners know what they should do but struggle with how to do it.

This collection emerged from that practical need. Over years of clinical practice, supervision, and training, I began documenting the specific phrases and responses that consistently created positive outcomes. I noticed patterns in the language that helped clients move from resistance to curiosity, from contemplation to commitment, from despair to hope. These weren't theoretical constructs but actual words spoken in real counseling sessions with measurable results.

The 500+ responses in this book represent field-tested language that has been refined through countless therapeutic encounters. Each phrase has been chosen not for its theoretical elegance but for its practical effectiveness in creating the kind of conversations that facilitate genuine change. They reflect the accumulated wisdom of practitioners who have learned what works through trial and error, success and failure, in the trenches of daily clinical work.

This is not another book about MI theory. Excellent theoretical texts already exist, and I encourage readers to study the foundational works by Jane Harlow (Motivational Interviewing for Beginners: A Step-by-Step Guide to Creating Meaningful Change), and other MI scholars. Instead, this is a practical companion—a response library that bridges the gap between knowing MI principles and applying them skillfully in real-world situations.

The organization follows the natural flow of therapeutic work, from opening sessions through the advanced techniques that experienced practitioners use to navigate complex situations. Each section provides multiple options because clients are unique individuals who respond differently to various approaches. What works with one person may fall flat with another, so having a repertoire of responses increases your chances of finding the right words for each unique situation.

These scripts are starting points, not rigid formulas. They're meant to be adapted to your personal style, your client's needs, and the specific context of your therapeutic relationship. The goal isn't to sound robotic or artificial but to have language available when you need it most—in those moments when the right words can make the difference between a session that goes nowhere and one that creates lasting change.

Mental health professionals work in an increasingly demanding environment. Caseloads are high, time is limited, and the complexity of client presentations continues to grow. Having ready access to effective therapeutic language can reduce preparation time, increase confidence in difficult situations, and ultimately improve outcomes for the people we serve.

This collection is offered in the spirit of mutual aid among helping professionals. Just as physicians share medical procedures and teachers share lesson plans, we can share the language tools that make our work more effective. The phrases in this book belong not to any individual practitioner but to the broader community of professionals committed to helping people change.

Use these responses wisely and adapt them thoughtfully. Let them serve as scaffolding while you develop your own authentic therapeutic voice. Most importantly, use them in service of your clients' goals and growth, not as techniques to demonstrate your skill or knowledge.

The ultimate measure of these scripts' value isn't how clever they sound but how well they help create the conditions where people feel safe enough to examine their lives honestly and motivated enough to make positive changes. If this collection helps you have more effective conversations with your clients, it has served its purpose.

Jane W. Harlow

Section I: Opening Scripts

The first words you speak in any counseling session carry tremendous weight. They set the tone, establish safety, and begin building the therapeutic alliance that makes change possible. In Motivational Interviewing, how you open creates the foundation for everything that follows.

Think about it: your client walks through that door carrying years of experiences with helping professionals. Maybe they've been lectured at, diagnosed, or had someone try to "fix" them. Maybe they're scared, defensive, or just going through the motions because someone else made them come. Those first few minutes can either confirm their worst fears about therapy or surprise them with something different.

The scripts in this section aren't magic formulas—they're conversation starters that honor the MI spirit while meeting people exactly where they are. Some clients need gentle warmth. Others respond to straightforward professionalism. A few require you to acknowledge the elephant in the room right away. The key is having options that feel authentic to you while serving your client's needs.

Chapter 1: First Sessions - 50 Ways to Begin

Walking into that first session, both you and your client are sizing each other up. They're wondering if you'll judge them, understand them, or waste their time. You're trying to create safety while gathering information. The pressure to get it "right" can feel intense.

But here's what I've learned after thousands of first sessions: there's no perfect opening. What matters is authenticity, curiosity, and a genuine desire to understand this person's world. The best openings feel conversational, not clinical. They invite rather than interrogate.

Creating Safety and Warmth

For the anxious or uncertain client:

1. "I'm glad you're here. I know it takes courage to walk through that door."
2. "Before we get started, I want you to know this is your time and your space. We'll go at whatever pace feels right for you."
3. "How are you feeling about being here today? It's completely normal to feel nervous."
4. "I'm wondering what it was like for you to make this appointment and actually show up today."
5. "First sessions can feel a little awkward. That's totally normal. We'll figure this out together."
6. "What would make this conversation most helpful for you today?"
7. "I imagine you might have some questions about how this works. What would you like to know?"

8. "There's no pressure to share anything you're not ready to talk about. We can start wherever feels comfortable."

Research consistently shows that perceived counselor warmth and acceptance in the first session predicts treatment engagement and outcomes (Lambert & Barley, 2001). These opening statements immediately communicate that this relationship will be different from other potentially judgmental encounters in the client's life.

For the quiet or withdrawn client:

9. "Sometimes it helps to start with something simple. How was your drive here today?"
10. "I notice you seem pretty quiet. That's perfectly fine. Some people like to take their time getting comfortable."
11. "No pressure to talk right away. Sometimes it takes a few minutes to settle in."
12. "I'm curious about what brought you here, but we can start wherever you'd like."
13. "Would it help if I told you a little bit about how I work, or would you rather jump into talking?"

Acknowledging Reality

Sometimes the most powerful opening acknowledges what's really happening in the room. These scripts address common concerns head-on.

When someone seems uncomfortable:

14. "This feels pretty formal, doesn't it? It doesn't have to stay that way."
15. "I'm sensing this might not be exactly how you wanted to spend your afternoon."
16. "You look like you're not entirely sure what to expect. Want to talk about that?"

17. "If you're thinking this is going to be one of those sessions where someone analyzes everything you say, you can relax. That's not my style."
18. "I get the feeling you might have some concerns about counseling. Most people do."

When acknowledging first-time therapy experiences:

19. "Is this your first time doing something like this? What has that been like for you?"
20. "I'm wondering if you have any ideas about therapy from movies or TV that might not match reality."
21. "Sometimes people come in expecting to lie on a couch and talk about their childhood. We can do that if you want, but we don't have to."
22. "Have you ever talked to a counselor before? How was that experience for you?"

The Curious Approach

Genuine curiosity is one of the most disarming and engaging qualities you can bring to a first session. These openings invite storytelling rather than symptom reporting.

Open-ended curiosity starters:

23. "I'd love to hear your story. Where would you like to begin?"
24. "What's been going on in your world that made you think counseling might be helpful?"
25. "Help me understand what life has been like for you lately."
26. "I'm curious about what's been on your mind recently."
27. "What's the most important thing you'd like me to know about you?"
28. "If you were going to catch me up on your life, where would you start?"
29. "What's been the biggest challenge you've been facing?"
30. "Tell me about a typical day in your life right now."

Miller and Rollnick (2013) emphasize that genuine curiosity communicates respect and helps clients feel heard rather than interrogated. This approach immediately shifts the dynamic from evaluation to collaboration.

The Practical Opener

Some clients appreciate a straightforward, business-like approach that focuses on goals and outcomes.

Goal-oriented beginnings:

31. "What would you like to be different in your life as a result of our work together?"
32. "If counseling goes well for you, how will you know? What will be different?"
33. "What's your hope for these sessions?"
34. "What would need to happen today for you to leave feeling like this was time well spent?"
35. "I'm wondering what success would look like for you in counseling."
36. "What's the main thing you'd like to work on?"
37. "If you could change one thing about your current situation, what would it be?"

When time is limited:

38. "We have about 50 minutes together today. How can we make the best use of that time?"
39. "I want to make sure we focus on what's most important to you. What should we prioritize?"
40. "What's the most pressing thing on your mind right now?"

The Collaborative Approach

These openings immediately establish the client as the expert on their own life while positioning you as a curious guide.

Partnership-focused openings:

41. "I'm here to help, but you're the expert on your own life. What do you think I should know?"
42. "My job is to listen and ask good questions. Your job is to be honest about what's really going on. Sound fair?"
43. "I have some experience with what people struggle with, but you're the only expert on what it's like to be you."
44. "I'm hoping we can figure this out together. What information would be most helpful for me to have?"
45. "You know yourself better than anyone. What do you think would be most helpful for us to talk about?"

Special Situation Openings

When someone was referred by another professional:

46. "Dr. Johnson mentioned she thought counseling might be helpful. What was that conversation like for you?"
47. "Your physician suggested we meet. How do you feel about that recommendation?"

When there's been a significant life event:

48. "I understand you've been through something really difficult recently. How are you holding up?"
49. "Sounds like there have been some major changes in your life. What's that been like?"

The universal backup:

50. "So... here we are. What brings you in today?"

Sometimes the simplest approach is the most effective. This final opening works in almost any situation because it's completely open-ended while acknowledging the shared reality that you're both here for a reason.

Making Your Choice

Not every opening will fit every client or feel natural coming from you. The goal isn't to memorize all 50 options but to have enough variety that you can respond authentically to whoever walks through your door.

Watch for nonverbal cues. A client who sits on the edge of their chair might need reassurance about safety. Someone who immediately starts talking might respond better to curious follow-up questions than lengthy explanations about the process. The person who looks around the room nervously might appreciate acknowledgment of their discomfort.

Remember, these openings are invitations, not interrogations. If one approach doesn't land well, you can always shift. "That question seemed to throw you off. Let me try a different way..." shows flexibility and responsiveness that clients appreciate.

The most important thing about any opening is that it comes from a genuine place of curiosity and care. Clients can sense authenticity, and they respond to it. When you're truly interested in understanding their experience, almost any words will work.

Chapter 2: Returning Clients - Re-engagement Phrases

The second session tells you everything about whether your first meeting worked. Some clients bounce through the door eager to continue. Others show up but seem distant or guarded. A few arrive looking like they'd rather be anywhere else. How you handle these different energies can make or break the therapeutic relationship.

Returning sessions require a different kind of attention than first meetings. You're not starting from scratch, but you're also not picking up exactly where you left off. Life happened between sessions. Your client had time to process, worry, doubt, or get excited about what you discussed. They might have tried something new or retreated back into old patterns.

The phrases in this chapter help you read the room and respond appropriately. They acknowledge the space between sessions while creating a bridge back into productive conversation.

Assessing Where They Are

Universal check-ins:

1. "How has your week been since we talked?"
2. "What's been on your mind since our last session?"
3. "How are you feeling about being back here today?"
4. "What's different for you today compared to last time?"
5. "I'm curious how you've been processing what we talked about."
6. "How did the time between sessions go for you?"

These simple openings give clients permission to share whatever is most present for them without making assumptions about their experience.

When They've Made Progress

Some clients return with visible positive changes or excited updates about progress they've made.

Celebrating forward movement:

7. "You seem different today. What's shifted for you?"
8. "I'm noticing something lighter about you. What's been going well?"
9. "Tell me about the changes you've been making."
10. "It sounds like some things have been moving in a positive direction."
11. "What's been working for you since we last met?"
12. "You look like someone who has good news to share."
13. "I can see something has changed. Walk me through what's been happening."
14. "What are you most proud of from this past week?"

Prochaska and Norcross (2018) note that acknowledging and amplifying client progress, however small, increases motivation and self-efficacy. These responses help clients recognize their own agency in creating change.

When they've tried something new:

15. "How did that experiment go that we talked about?"
16. "What was it like to try something different?"
17. "You took a risk. How did that feel?"
18. "What did you learn about yourself by trying that?"
19. "Even trying was a big step. What was that experience like?"

When They Seem Stuck or Discouraged

Not every return session brings good news. Sometimes clients come back feeling defeated, having had a difficult week, or questioning whether counseling is helping.

Normalizing difficulty:

20. "Sounds like it's been a tough week. What's been the hardest part?"
21. "Some weeks are just hard. You still showed up here, though."
22. "It takes courage to come back when things aren't going well."
23. "What's been weighing on you since we last talked?"
24. "I'm glad you're here, especially when it's been difficult."
25. "How can we make sense of what's been happening?"
26. "What would be most helpful to focus on today?"

When they express doubt about counseling:

27. "You seem less sure about this process today. What's changed?"
28. "I'm sensing some hesitation. Tell me more about that."
29. "It sounds like you're questioning whether this is helping."
30. "What would need to be different for this to feel more useful?"
31. "Sometimes counseling feels slow. Is that part of what you're experiencing?"
32. "What's making you wonder if this is worth your time?"

Research on therapeutic alliance emphasizes that addressing ruptures or doubts directly often strengthens the relationship (Safran & Kraus, 2014). These responses invite honest conversation about the process itself.

When They Seem Distant or Withdrawn

Some clients return but seem less engaged than they were initially. They might give shorter answers, seem distracted, or appear to be going through the motions.

Gentle invitations back into connection:

33. "You seem quieter today. What's going on for you?"
34. "I'm noticing you seem a little more reserved than last time."
35. "Something feels different in the room today. What are you experiencing?"
36. "You look like your mind is somewhere else. What's taking up your mental space?"
37. "I'm getting the sense that part of you doesn't want to be here today."
38. "You seem more guarded than when we first met. What's that about?"
39. "Is there something about last session that didn't sit well with you?"

When they seem to be holding back:

40. "What's the thing you're not telling me?"
41. "There seems to be more under the surface. What's happening internally?"
42. "You look like you want to say something but aren't sure if you should."
43. "What would you say if you knew it was completely safe?"
44. "I have the feeling there's something important you're hesitating to share."

When They've Had a Crisis or Setback

Sometimes clients return after experiencing a significant challenge, relapse, or crisis situation.

Responding to crisis or setback:

45. "What happened? Start wherever you need to."
46. "That sounds incredibly difficult. How are you managing?"
47. "You made it through something really hard and you're here. That says something about your strength."
48. "Crisis moments can teach us things. What are you learning about yourself?"
49. "How can we use what happened to move forward?"
50. "What do you need most right now in terms of support?"
51. "You've survived difficult things before. What helped you get through those times?"

When they've experienced a relapse:

52. "Setbacks are part of the process for most people. What can we learn from what happened?"
53. "You're here talking about it, which means you haven't given up."
54. "What was different about the circumstances that led to this?"
55. "How do you want to move forward from here?"

Transitional Phrases

These phrases help move from the check-in phase into deeper work while honoring whatever energy or mood the client brings.

Moving into the session's work:

56. "What feels most important to focus on today?"
57. "Given everything you've shared, where should we put our energy?"
58. "What would make today's session most valuable for you?"
59. "I'm hearing several things. Which one feels most pressing?"
60. "What's calling for your attention right now?"

When building on previous sessions:

61. "That connects to what we were talking about last time."

62. "I'm seeing a pattern we've discussed before. What do you make of that?"
63. "This reminds me of something you said last week. Do you see the connection?"
64. "How does this relate to the goal you mentioned working toward?"

Reading the Nonverbals

The returning client's body language, energy level, and general demeanor tell you as much as their words. Someone who sits in the same chair as last time might be getting comfortable. A client who chooses a different seat might be signaling a need for change or distance.

Pay attention to timing. The client who arrives early might be eager to work. Someone who shows up right on time might be managing their ambivalence by limiting their exposure. The person who arrives a few minutes late might be testing boundaries or dealing with avoidance.

Energy matters too. High energy might indicate breakthrough insights or anxiety. Low energy could signal depression, exhaustion, or resistance. Your job isn't to match their energy but to meet it with curiosity and appropriate response.

The Art of Pacing

Returning sessions require sensitivity to pacing. Some clients need time to settle back into the therapeutic space. Others want to jump right into current concerns. The phrases in this chapter give you options for both approaches.

When in doubt, let the client lead. "Where would you like to start today?" puts them in control while showing your flexibility. If they seem uncertain, you can offer gentle structure: "Would it help if we started with how things have been since we last talked?"

Remember that every return session is both a continuation and a new beginning. You're building on what came before while remaining open to whatever emerges today. The strongest therapeutic relationships balance consistency with responsiveness, honoring both the process and the person.

Chapter 3: Reluctant Participants - Court-Ordered and Mandated Clients

Let's be honest about something right up front: nobody wants to be told they have to go to counseling. When someone sits across from you because a judge, employer, or family member said they had no choice, you're dealing with a completely different dynamic than voluntary counseling.

These clients often arrive with their defenses up and their expectations low. They might be angry, resentful, or just planning to sit there and wait out the required sessions. Some see you as part of the system that's controlling them. Others have given up hope that anything will change anyway.

But here's what I've learned working with thousands of mandated clients: resistance isn't personal, and it isn't permanent. Underneath that armor is usually someone who's been hurt, disappointed, or failed by systems before. They're protecting themselves the only way they know how.

The scripts in this chapter help you work with resistance instead of against it. They acknowledge reality, respect autonomy even within constraints, and create space for authentic change to occur.

Acknowledging the Elephant

The worst thing you can do with a mandated client is pretend they're there voluntarily. The elephant in the room needs to be named early and directly.

Direct acknowledgment:

1. "I understand you're here because someone else said you had to be. How does that sit with you?"
2. "This probably isn't how you wanted to spend your time today."
3. "I'm guessing being required to come here doesn't feel great."
4. "Let's talk about the fact that you didn't exactly choose to be here."
5. "Most people don't love being told they have to do counseling. How are you feeling about it?"
6. "I know you're here because of what the court/judge/employer decided. What's that been like for you?"

Normalizing their response:

7. "It makes complete sense that you'd feel frustrated about having to be here."
8. "I'd probably feel the same way if someone told me I had to do something I didn't want to do."
9. "Being mandated to counseling can feel pretty invasive. Is that part of what you're experiencing?"
10. "It's normal to feel resistant when choice gets taken away."

Research on psychological reactance theory shows that when people feel their freedom is threatened, they naturally push back (Brehm & Brehm, 2013). Acknowledging this response reduces defensiveness and creates space for collaboration.

Exploring Their Perspective

Once you've acknowledged the involuntary nature of their attendance, you can begin exploring their experience and perspective.

Understanding their viewpoint:

11. "Help me understand how you see this situation."

12. "What's your take on why you were referred here?"
13. "From your perspective, what do other people think needs to change?"
14. "What's it like to have other people making decisions about what you need?"
15. "I'm curious about your thoughts on the concerns that brought you here."
16. "What do you think about the idea that counseling might be helpful?"

Exploring the mandate:

17. "Tell me about the situation that led to this requirement."
18. "What do you understand about what you need to accomplish here?"
19. "How long are you required to come, and what does compliance look like?"
20. "What happens if you complete these sessions? What happens if you don't?"
21. "Who else is involved in monitoring your participation here?"

Finding Their Motivation

Even mandated clients have reasons they might want things to be different in their lives. Your job is to find those reasons and connect them to the work.

Looking for intrinsic motivation:

22. "Setting aside what other people want, is there anything you'd like to see change in your life?"
23. "If you could wave a magic wand and fix one thing about your current situation, what would it be?"
24. "What would your life look like if all these problems just went away?"
25. "Is there anything about your current situation that bothers you?"

26. "What do you miss about how things used to be before all this started?"
27. "If you weren't required to be here, is there anything you might want help with anyway?"

Connecting consequences to their values:

28. "How is all this legal/work/family stuff affecting the things that matter to you?"
29. "What's been the hardest part about dealing with all these requirements and restrictions?"
30. "How has this situation impacted your relationships with people you care about?"
31. "What freedoms or opportunities have you lost because of what's happened?"

Miller and Rollnick (2013) emphasize that even in mandated situations, clients retain autonomy over their internal responses and future choices. Finding genuine motivation increases engagement and improves outcomes.

Working with Anger and Resentment

Many mandated clients carry significant anger about their situation, the system, or the people who referred them. This anger needs to be acknowledged and worked with, not ignored or minimized.

Validating anger:

32. "You sound really angry about all this. That makes sense."
33. "I can hear how frustrated you are with the whole situation."
34. "It sounds like you feel like people are trying to control you."
35. "Being angry about losing choices is completely understandable."
36. "You have every right to feel upset about how this all happened."

Channeling anger productively:

37. "That anger you're feeling - could it be useful energy for making some changes?"
38. "What would you want to say to the people who put you in this situation?"
39. "How do you usually handle feeling this angry?"
40. "What would it look like to use that frustration to fuel something positive?"

Establishing Clear Boundaries and Expectations

Mandated clients need to understand exactly what's expected of them and what they can expect from you. Clarity reduces anxiety and resistance.

Setting expectations:

41. "Let me be clear about what I'm required to report and what stays between us."
42. "Here's what compliance looks like from my perspective, and here's where you have choices."
43. "I'm not here to judge whether what you did was right or wrong. I'm here to help you figure out how to move forward."
44. "My job is to provide the sessions that were required. Your job is to show up. Everything else is up to you."
45. "You get to decide how much you participate beyond just being physically present."

Addressing confidentiality concerns:

46. "I understand you might be worried about what I'll tell other people. Let's talk about how that works."
47. "What are your concerns about privacy and confidentiality?"
48. "You have the right to know what information gets shared and with whom."
49. "How can we work together within these reporting requirements?"

Creating Choice Within Constraints

Even though mandated clients must attend sessions, they still have choices about how they engage. Highlighting these choices can restore some sense of autonomy.

Emphasizing remaining choices:

50. "You have to be here, but you get to choose how you want to use this time."
51. "While you can't control that you're required to come, you can control what you get out of it."
52. "What would make these mandatory sessions feel less like a waste of your time?"
53. "How do you want to approach these sessions? We can do the minimum required, or we can try to make them actually helpful."
54. "You're going to be here anyway. What would make it worthwhile for you?"

Collaborative planning:

55. "What would you like to focus on during our time together?"
56. "How can we make these sessions work for both of us?"
57. "What would success look like from your perspective?"
58. "If you're stuck doing this, how can we make it as useful as possible?"

Dealing with Resistance and Testing

Mandated clients often test boundaries and express resistance in various ways. How you respond to these tests often determines whether a working relationship develops.

When they're silent or minimal:

59. "Silence is one way to handle being somewhere you don't want to be."

60. "You don't have to talk if you're not ready. Your choice."
61. "Sometimes people need time to decide if this is going to be safe."
62. "What would need to happen for you to feel comfortable talking more?"

When they challenge your authority or expertise:

63. "It sounds like you don't think I can help you. Tell me more about that."
64. "You're right that I don't know what it's like to be in your situation."
65. "What would I need to understand about your life for this to be useful?"
66. "You're the expert on your own experience. I'm just here to listen and ask questions."

Building Alliance Over Time

With mandated clients, the therapeutic alliance often develops slowly and requires consistent demonstration of respect and authenticity.

Demonstrating respect:

67. "I respect that you're handling a difficult situation."
68. "You're dealing with a lot of pressure from different directions."
69. "It takes strength to get through what you're going through."
70. "You're here even though you don't want to be. That says something about your character."

Showing authenticity:

71. "I'm not going to pretend this is normal counseling. We both know it's not."
72. "I can't make your legal/work problems go away, but maybe we can figure out how to make them more manageable."

73. "I'm not here to fix you because I don't think you're broken."
74. "My job isn't to convince you that what happened was wrong. You already know how you feel about it."

The Long Game

Working with mandated clients requires patience and a long-term perspective. Change rarely happens quickly, and trust develops slowly. Some clients will remain resistant throughout the required sessions but might seek help voluntarily later when they're ready.

Your role isn't to break down their resistance but to plant seeds that might grow when conditions are right. Sometimes the most important thing you do is simply treat them with dignity and respect during a difficult time in their life.

Remember that many mandated clients have had negative experiences with authority figures and helping professionals. You might be the first person in their recent experience who doesn't try to control, judge, or change them. That alone can be powerful.

The goal isn't to make them grateful for being mandated to counseling. The goal is to help them find whatever motivation and resources they need to create positive change in their lives, even within the constraints they're facing.

These opening scripts set the foundation for everything that follows in your MI practice. Whether someone walks through your door eagerly, reluctantly, or somewhere in between, you now have language that meets them exactly where they are.

The next section moves into the core responses that make up the heart of Motivational Interviewing—the reflections, affirmations, and summaries that create the conversational dance of change. But everything starts with how you begin. When you master these opening moments, you create the safety and curiosity that makes transformation possible.

Part II: Core MI Responses

If opening scripts are the foundation of MI, then core responses are the walls and framework that build the therapeutic relationship. These aren't just techniques you memorize—they're ways of being with another person that communicate deep respect, genuine curiosity, and unwavering belief in their capacity for change.

The four core responses in this section form the backbone of every MI conversation: simple reflections that mirror back what you hear, complex reflections that add depth and meaning, affirmations that highlight strengths and efforts, and summary statements that weave everything together. Master these, and you'll have the tools to create the kind of conversations that help people talk themselves into change.

Chapter 4: Simple Reflections - 75 Versatile Phrases

Simple reflections are the bread and butter of Motivational Interviewing. They're deceptively straightforward—you listen to what someone says and reflect it back in slightly different words. But don't let the simplicity fool you. A well-timed simple reflection can be more powerful than the most brilliant interpretation or insight.

Think about the last time someone really listened to you. Not the kind of listening where they're waiting for their turn to talk, but the kind where they hang on every word and reflect back what they heard. How did that feel? Most people say it feels validating, clarifying, even healing. That's the power of simple reflections.

Simple reflections serve multiple purposes in MI. They slow down the conversation, giving both you and your client time to process what's being said. They demonstrate that you're truly listening, not just waiting to give advice. Most importantly, they give clients the chance to hear their own thoughts reflected back, which often helps them understand themselves better.

The Art of Almost Repeating

A simple reflection isn't parroting back exactly what someone said. That feels mechanical and annoying. Instead, it's offering back the essence of what you heard using slightly different words. The goal is to capture not just the content but the emotional tone underneath.

Basic feeling reflections:

1. "You're feeling frustrated about this."

2. "That sounds really disappointing."
3. "You seem pretty angry about what happened."
4. "This has been weighing on you."
5. "You're worried about how this might turn out."
6. "That must have been scary."
7. "You sound relieved about that decision."
8. "This feels overwhelming right now."
9. "You're excited about this possibility."
10. "That's been really stressful for you."

Research consistently shows that accurate empathy, demonstrated through reflective listening, is one of the strongest predictors of positive therapeutic outcomes across all approaches (Elliott et al., 2011). These basic reflections communicate that you understand both the content and emotional impact of what your client is sharing.

Content reflections:

11. "So what you're saying is..."
12. "It sounds like the main issue is..."
13. "You're dealing with multiple problems at once."
14. "The timing of all this has been particularly difficult."
15. "You've been trying several different approaches."
16. "This pattern has been going on for a while."
17. "You're seeing some connections between these events."
18. "The pressure from different directions is intense."
19. "You've got a lot on your plate right now."
20. "This situation keeps changing."

Reflecting Ambivalence

One of the most important skills in MI is reflecting the natural ambivalence that most people feel about change. Simple reflections help clients explore both sides of their internal conflicts.

Two-sided reflections:

21. "Part of you wants to change, and part of you isn't sure."

22. "You're torn between staying safe and taking a risk."
23. "On one hand you see the benefits, but on the other hand you're concerned about the cost."
24. "You want things to be different, but change feels scary."
25. "You know what you should do, but doing it feels impossible."
26. "You're tired of the way things are, but you're also afraid of making them worse."
27. "You see the logic in what people are telling you, but emotionally it doesn't feel right."

Reflecting internal conflict:

28. "You're really struggling with this decision."
29. "This feels like an impossible choice."
30. "You're getting mixed messages from different parts of yourself."
31. "Your head and your heart seem to be saying different things."
32. "You feel pulled in opposite directions."
33. "This decision would be easier if you only had to consider one factor."

Continuing the Paragraph

This technique involves picking up where your client left off, as if you're finishing their thought. It's particularly useful when someone trails off or seems to be searching for words.

Continuation reflections:

34. "And when that happened, you felt..."
35. "So then you found yourself..."
36. "Which left you wondering..."
37. "And that made you realize..."
38. "So now you're thinking..."
39. "Which brings up the question of..."
40. "And underneath all that, you're..."

Reflecting Values and Meaning

Simple reflections can highlight what matters most to your clients, helping them connect with their deeper motivations.

Value-based reflections:

41. "Being a good parent really matters to you."
42. "Your independence is something you value highly."
43. "Honesty in relationships is non-negotiable for you."
44. "You take your responsibilities seriously."
45. "Family comes first in your priorities."
46. "You want to be someone you can respect."
47. "Making a difference matters more than making money."
48. "You value authenticity over appearance."

Meaning-making reflections:

49. "This experience taught you something important about yourself."
50. "You're starting to see a bigger picture."
51. "There's a lesson in all this for you."
52. "This connects to something deeper you're working on."
53. "You're finding meaning in what happened."

Reflecting Change Talk

When clients express any desire, ability, reason, or need for change, simple reflections can amplify these statements and encourage more exploration.

Desire reflections:

54. "You really want things to be different."
55. "You wish you could handle this better."
56. "You'd like to feel more in control."
57. "You want to be the kind of person who..."
58. "You're hoping for a better outcome."

Ability reflections:

59. "You think you could do this if..."
60. "You've had success with similar challenges before."
61. "You're capable of more than you sometimes believe."
62. "You have the skills to figure this out."
63. "You're stronger than you give yourself credit for."

Reason reflections:

64. "The benefits of changing are becoming clearer to you."
65. "You can see how this would improve your life."
66. "The cost of staying the same is getting too high."
67. "You're recognizing the impact on people you care about."

Need reflections:

68. "Something has to change."
69. "You can't keep going like this."
70. "This situation requires action."
71. "The status quo isn't working anymore."

Miller and Rollnick (2013) identify these four types of change talk as particularly important to recognize and reflect. When clients hear their own change talk reflected back, they often elaborate and strengthen their commitment to change.

Advanced Simple Reflections

These reflections add subtle depth while maintaining the simplicity that makes this technique so powerful.

Slightly amplified reflections:

72. "This has been incredibly difficult for you." (when they said it was "hard")
73. "You're absolutely exhausted by all this." (when they said they were "tired")

74. "You're really passionate about this issue." (when they expressed strong concern)
75. "This means everything to you." (when they indicated something was important)

Getting the Tone Right

The way you deliver a simple reflection matters as much as the words you choose. Your tone should be curious and slightly tentative, as if you're checking your understanding rather than making a definitive statement. Think of it as offering a gentle mirror rather than making a pronouncement.

The inflection pattern makes a difference too. Ending with a slightly rising tone (like a question) invites confirmation or correction. Ending with a falling tone (like a statement) can feel more definitive and might shut down further exploration.

Watch for your client's response to your reflections. If they say "exactly" or "that's right" and then elaborate, you're on target. If they correct you or seem confused, adjust your approach. The goal isn't to be perfect but to stay close enough to their experience that they feel heard and understood.

When Simple Reflections Go Wrong

Sometimes simple reflections miss the mark. Maybe you focus on content when the emotion is more important. Maybe you reflect back exactly what they said instead of adding any new perspective. Maybe your timing is off, interrupting their flow instead of encouraging it.

Don't worry about getting every reflection perfect. The attempt to understand is often more important than perfect accuracy. When you miss, pay attention to how your client corrects you. Their corrections often contain the most important information.

Some clients will test your listening by sharing something and then waiting to see if you really heard them. Others will correct your reflections as a way of maintaining control in the conversation. Both responses are normal and workable.

Building Reflection Skills

Like any skill, simple reflections improve with practice. Start by paying attention to the feeling words your clients use. Notice when they express ambivalence or internal conflict. Listen for values and what matters most to them.

Practice varying your reflection stems. Instead of always starting with "It sounds like...", try "You're feeling..." or "So for you..." or "What I'm hearing is...". The more natural and varied your reflections sound, the more effective they'll be.

Pay attention to what happens after your reflections. Do clients elaborate? Correct you? Go deeper? These responses tell you whether you're tracking with their experience or missing something important.

Most importantly, reflect from a place of genuine curiosity rather than technique. When you're truly interested in understanding your client's experience, the words will usually come naturally.

The Deeper Purpose

Simple reflections do more than just demonstrate good listening. They slow down conversations that might otherwise rush toward premature solutions. They help clients process their own thoughts by hearing them reflected back. They create space for emotions to be acknowledged and explored.

In our advice-giving culture, simply reflecting what someone says can feel revolutionary. It communicates that their experience matters, their perspective has value, and they don't need to be fixed or changed immediately. That space to be heard and understood often becomes the foundation for genuine change.

Chapter 5: Complex Reflections - Advanced Formulations

While simple reflections mirror back what clients say, complex reflections add depth, meaning, and new perspective. They're like taking a photograph and adjusting the focus, brightness, or angle to reveal details that weren't immediately visible. These reflections require more skill and intuition, but they can unlock insights that simple reflections can't reach.

Complex reflections are where artistry meets technique in MI. They require you to listen not just to what's being said, but to what's underneath—the fears, hopes, values, and meanings that drive behavior. When done skillfully, they help clients see their situations from new angles and discover motivations they didn't know they had.

The risk with complex reflections is overstepping—adding interpretations that come from your agenda rather than their material. The goal isn't to show how clever you are or to push clients in a particular direction. It's to offer perspectives that help them understand themselves more deeply and move toward their own conclusions about change.

Amplified Reflections

These reflections take what a client says and intensify it slightly, helping them recognize the full impact or importance of their experience.

Emotional amplification:

1. "This isn't just frustrating—it's absolutely maddening for you."
2. "You're not just worried—you're genuinely frightened about what might happen."
3. "This doesn't just matter to you—it's at the core of who you are."
4. "You're not just disappointed—you feel completely betrayed."
5. "This isn't just difficult—it's been devastating."
6. "You're not just tired—you're completely exhausted by all of this."
7. "This isn't just a setback—it feels like everything is falling apart."

Amplified reflections can help clients recognize feelings they've been minimizing or avoiding. Sometimes people need permission to acknowledge the full weight of their experiences.

Consequence amplification:

8. "If this continues, you could lose everything that matters to you."
9. "This isn't just affecting you—it's hurting the people you love most."
10. "The cost of not changing is becoming unbearable."
11. "This pattern is destroying your self-respect."
12. "You're not just risking your job—you're risking your entire career."

Double-Sided Reflections

These reflections capture both sides of a client's ambivalence in a single statement, highlighting the internal tension they're experiencing.

Classic double-sided reflections:

13. "You want to quit drinking because it's causing problems, but you also worry about losing the one thing that helps you relax."
14. "Part of you knows you need to leave this relationship, and part of you still loves him and hopes things will change."
15. "You're excited about the possibility of a new career, but you're also terrified of giving up the security you have now."
16. "You want to be honest with your parents about who you are, but you're afraid of losing their love and support."
17. "You know exercise would help you feel better, but right now you barely have energy to get through each day."

Value conflict reflections:

18. "Your desire for independence conflicts with your need for security."
19. "You value honesty, but you also want to protect people from painful truths."
20. "Being a good employee matters to you, but so does having time for your family."
21. "You want to be authentic, but you also need to be accepted."

Research on decisional balance shows that acknowledging both sides of ambivalence helps clients work through internal conflicts more effectively than focusing on only one side (Janis & Mann, 1977). These reflections normalize the complexity of human motivation.

Metaphorical Reflections

Sometimes a metaphor or analogy can capture a client's experience more powerfully than direct description.

Life situation metaphors:

22. "It sounds like you're stuck between a rock and a hard place."

23. "You feel like you're drowning, and everyone keeps telling you to swim harder."
24. "It's like you're driving with the brakes on—part of you wants to move forward, but part of you is holding back."
25. "You're carrying the weight of the world on your shoulders."
26. "It feels like you're walking on eggshells all the time."
27. "You're at a crossroads, and every path seems to have risks."
28. "It's like being in a storm where you can't see the horizon."

Process metaphors:

29. "You're trying to fill a bucket that has holes in the bottom."
30. "It's like you're speaking a different language than everyone else."
31. "You feel like you're swimming against the current."
32. "It's as if you're wearing a mask that you can't take off."
33. "You're running on empty, but everyone expects you to keep going."

Reframes and New Perspectives

These reflections offer alternative ways of understanding a situation, often highlighting strengths or possibilities that weren't initially apparent.

Strength-based reframes:

34. "What you're calling stubbornness might actually be persistence and determination."
35. "Your sensitivity, which you see as a weakness, might be one of your greatest gifts."
36. "The fact that you care so much shows how deeply you love."
37. "Your perfectionism comes from wanting to do things well."
38. "Your caution isn't cowardice—it's wisdom from past experiences."
39. "What others might see as giving up, you're seeing as choosing your battles."

Developmental reframes:

40. "This crisis might be pushing you toward growth you wouldn't have chosen but needed."
41. "What feels like falling apart might actually be breaking open."
42. "This setback could be redirecting you toward something better."
43. "Sometimes we have to lose what we thought we wanted to find what we actually need."
44. "This difficult period might be teaching you something important about yourself."

Reflecting Unspoken Material

These reflections address what clients haven't said directly but that seems present in their story or manner.

Underlying emotions:

45. "Beneath all that anger, I'm hearing a lot of hurt."
46. "Under the anxiety, there seems to be excitement about this possibility."
47. "Behind the guilt, I sense some anger about how you've been treated."
48. "Underneath the sadness, there might be some relief."
49. "Beyond the fear, I'm hearing hope."

Hidden motivations:

50. "It sounds like proving yourself to others has become more important than taking care of yourself."
51. "Maybe the real issue isn't whether you can change, but whether you deserve to be happy."
52. "This might be less about the specific problem and more about feeling in control of your life."
53. "Perhaps what you're really searching for is a sense of meaning and purpose."

54. "The underlying question seems to be whether you can trust yourself to make good decisions."

Reflections That Evoke Values

These reflections help clients connect with what matters most to them, which often provides motivation for change.

Core value reflections:

55. "Being a good parent isn't just what you do—it's who you are."
56. "Living with integrity matters more to you than being comfortable."
57. "You'd rather struggle with the truth than be content with a lie."
58. "Freedom and independence are worth almost any sacrifice to you."
59. "You need your life to have meaning, not just success."
60. "Authenticity is more important to you than approval."

Value-behavior discrepancy reflections:

61. "There's a gap between who you want to be and how you're living right now."
62. "Your actions aren't matching your values, and that's eating at you."
63. "You're living someone else's definition of success instead of your own."
64. "The person you're becoming isn't the person you admire."
65. "Your current choices are taking you away from what matters most."

Reflections That Highlight Change Process

These reflections draw attention to movement, growth, or readiness for change that clients might not fully recognize.

Process reflections:

66. "You're in a different place today than you were six months ago."
67. "Something is shifting inside you, even if you can't name it yet."
68. "You're asking different questions now than when we first started talking."
69. "The fact that you're here shows you're ready for something to change."
70. "You're seeing patterns now that were invisible to you before."
71. "You're starting to trust your own judgment again."

Readiness reflections:

72. "You sound like someone who's getting ready to make a move."
73. "There's an urgency in your voice that wasn't there before."
74. "You're done making excuses and ready to face reality."
75. "Something inside you is saying 'enough is enough.'"

The Timing of Complex Reflections

Complex reflections require careful timing. Offered too early in a relationship, they can feel invasive or presumptuous. Offered at the right moment, they can provide breakthrough insights that accelerate change.

Watch for moments when clients seem to be searching for words, when they pause thoughtfully, or when they express confusion about their own reactions. These are often opportunities for complex reflections that add clarity or depth.

Pay attention to your client's response to complex reflections. If they light up and say "exactly!" or "I never thought of it that way," you've probably hit something important. If they look confused or correct you, you may have overreached or misunderstood their experience.

Building Complex Reflection Skills

Developing skill with complex reflections requires practice listening for subtext and developing comfort with uncertainty. You're making educated guesses about your client's internal experience, which means you'll sometimes be wrong.

Start by noticing discrepancies between what clients say and how they say it. Pay attention to energy shifts, body language changes, and emotional undertones. These often point toward material that might benefit from complex reflection.

Practice using tentative language: "I wonder if..." "It seems like maybe..." "I'm getting the sense that..." This invites collaboration rather than imposing your interpretations.

Most importantly, stay curious rather than clever. The goal isn't to impress clients with your insights but to offer perspectives that help them understand themselves better.

The Power and Responsibility

Complex reflections can be tremendously powerful tools for helping clients see their situations from new angles and connect with deeper motivations. They can also be invasive or harmful if used carelessly.

Always check your motivations when offering complex reflections. Are you trying to help the client understand themselves better, or are you pushing your own agenda? Are you offering a perspective that serves them, or one that makes you feel skilled?

The best complex reflections feel like gifts—they offer something valuable that clients can accept, reject, or modify as they see fit. They never force conclusions but invite exploration. When used skillfully, they help clients become the authors of their own change stories rather than passive recipients of your interpretations.

Chapter 6: Affirmation Arsenal - 100 Strength-Spotting Statements

Most people walk into counseling focused on what's wrong with them. They've usually been thinking about their problems, failures, and shortcomings for a while before they seek help. They expect you to focus on those same deficits. Affirmations do something radical—they shine a light on what's right, what's working, and what's possible.

But affirmations in MI aren't cheerleading or false positivity. They're not about telling people they're wonderful when they feel terrible. Real affirmations recognize genuine strengths, efforts, and positive qualities that clients possess but may not see or value. They're about helping people recognize their own resources for change.

The challenge is learning to spot strengths that are hiding in plain sight. When someone tells you about their failures, can you see the values that drove their efforts? When they describe their struggles, can you recognize the courage it takes to keep trying? When they criticize themselves, can you hear the high standards that motivate them?

Effort and Persistence Affirmations

Some of the most powerful affirmations recognize the energy and determination people put into trying to change, even when their efforts haven't been successful.

Recognizing effort:

1. "You've been working really hard at this."

2. "The effort you're putting in shows how much this matters to you."
3. "You haven't given up, even when it would have been easier to quit."
4. "You keep trying different approaches until you find what works."
5. "The persistence you're showing is remarkable."
6. "You're not accepting defeat easily."
7. "You're willing to keep experimenting until you find a solution."
8. "Your determination is impressive."
9. "You've shown incredible staying power through all this."
10. "You're fighting for what matters to you."

Persistence through setbacks:

11. "You get knocked down, but you keep getting back up."
12. "Each setback teaches you something, and you apply what you learn."
13. "You're not letting failures define you."
14. "You see setbacks as information, not evidence that you should quit."
15. "You bounce back from disappointments faster than most people."
16. "Your resilience in the face of challenges is inspiring."
17. "You've survived difficult situations before, and you're doing it again."

Courage and Risk-Taking Affirmations

Many positive changes require courage—the willingness to face fears, take risks, or do things differently. These affirmations recognize that bravery.

Acknowledging courage:

18. "It takes courage to look honestly at yourself like this."
19. "You're brave enough to face some uncomfortable truths."

20. "Asking for help requires real strength."
21. "You're willing to be vulnerable in service of growth."
22. "You're facing your fears instead of running from them."
23. "You're taking risks that could lead to positive change."
24. "You're choosing growth over comfort."
25. "You're brave enough to try something different."

Research shows that acknowledging client courage and risk-taking increases their willingness to continue making difficult changes (Snyder et al., 2000). These affirmations can provide fuel for continued effort.

Risk-taking recognition:

26. "You're willing to step outside your comfort zone."
27. "You took a chance, and that shows character."
28. "You're not playing it safe—you're playing to win."
29. "You'd rather risk failure than guarantee mediocrity."
30. "You're choosing possibility over security."

Values-Based Affirmations

These affirmations highlight the positive values and principles that guide a person's actions, even when those actions haven't led to desired outcomes.

Core values recognition:

31. "Your integrity matters more to you than convenience."
32. "You care deeply about doing the right thing."
33. "Being authentic is more important to you than being popular."
34. "You have a strong moral compass."
35. "You stand up for what you believe in."
36. "Your compassion for others is evident in how you talk about them."
37. "You hold yourself to high standards."
38. "You value honesty, even when it's difficult."

39. "You put others' needs ahead of your own comfort."
40. "You're committed to being a person of your word."

Relational values:

41. "Your love for your family drives everything you do."
42. "Being a good friend matters tremendously to you."
43. "You take your responsibilities to others seriously."
44. "You're willing to sacrifice for people you care about."
45. "You want to be someone others can count on."
46. "Your loyalty to people you love is unwavering."
47. "You invest in relationships that matter."

Self-Awareness Affirmations

These affirmations recognize a client's growing insight, self-understanding, or ability to reflect on their own experience.

Insight recognition:

48. "You have remarkable insight into yourself."
49. "You're very aware of your own patterns."
50. "You see connections that others might miss."
51. "You understand yourself better than most people understand themselves."
52. "Your self-reflection skills are impressive."
53. "You're honest about your own contributions to problems."
54. "You can step back and see the bigger picture."
55. "You have good judgment about people and situations."

Learning and growth:

56. "You learn from your mistakes instead of just regretting them."
57. "You're always working on becoming a better person."
58. "You're open to feedback and willing to change."
59. "You don't make the same mistake twice."
60. "You're curious about yourself and committed to growth."

61. "You turn experiences into wisdom."

Strength in Adversity Affirmations

These affirmations recognize how people handle difficult circumstances and what their responses reveal about their character.

Coping strength:

62. "You handle stress better than most people could."
63. "You find ways to keep going even when things get tough."
64. "Your ability to cope with adversity is remarkable."
65. "You maintain your sense of humor even in difficult times."
66. "You don't let circumstances defeat your spirit."
67. "You find strength you didn't know you had."
68. "You're tougher than you give yourself credit for."

Protective instincts:

69. "You're protective of people who matter to you."
70. "You shield others from your own pain."
71. "You put on a brave face so others don't have to worry."
72. "You take care of everyone else, even when you're struggling."
73. "Your instinct is to help others, even when you need help yourself."

Resourcefulness and Problem-Solving Affirmations

These recognize a person's creativity, adaptability, and ability to find solutions.

Creative problem-solving:

74. "You're incredibly resourceful when you need to be."
75. "You find creative solutions to complex problems."

76. "You think outside the box when conventional approaches don't work."
77. "You're adaptable and flexible when circumstances change."
78. "You make the best of whatever situation you're in."
79. "You're good at finding alternatives when plan A doesn't work."
80. "You have a talent for seeing opportunities others miss."

Communication and Relationship Affirmations

These affirmations recognize interpersonal strengths and communication skills.

Communication strengths:

81. "You express yourself clearly and thoughtfully."
82. "You're a good listener who really hears what people are saying."
83. "You have a gift for making people feel comfortable."
84. "You know how to connect with different types of people."
85. "You're skilled at reading between the lines."
86. "You have a way of bringing out the best in others."

Relationship building:

87. "People trust you because you're trustworthy."
88. "You create safe spaces for others to be authentic."
89. "You're the kind of person others turn to for support."
90. "You invest in relationships for the long term."
91. "You forgive others more easily than you forgive yourself."

Present Moment Affirmations

These affirmations recognize positive qualities or choices that are evident right now in the counseling session.

Current session strengths:

92. "You're being completely honest with me right now."
93. "You're not making excuses or blaming others."
94. "You're taking responsibility for your part in this."
95. "You're open to looking at this from different angles."
96. "You're willing to consider possibilities you haven't explored before."
97. "You're here doing the hard work of change."
98. "You're investing in your future by being here."
99. "You're choosing to face reality instead of avoiding it."
100. "Right now, you're exactly where you need to be to move forward."

Delivering Affirmations Effectively

The power of an affirmation lies not just in the words but in how and when you deliver it. Timing matters enormously. An affirmation offered right after someone shares something difficult can feel dismissive. An affirmation that follows a client's expression of self-doubt can feel perfectly timed and deeply meaningful.

Your tone should be genuine and matter-of-fact, not effusive or cheerleader-like. You're pointing out something real that you see, not trying to make someone feel better with false praise.

Specificity makes affirmations more powerful. Instead of saying "You're strong," try "The way you handled your daughter's crisis while dealing with your own problems shows incredible strength." The more specific you are, the more believable and impactful the affirmation becomes.

Avoiding Common Pitfalls

Not every positive comment is an effective affirmation. Avoid empty praise ("You're amazing"), comparative statements ("You're better than most people"), or affirmations that contradict the client's current experience ("You should feel proud when they clearly feel ashamed").

Be careful not to over-affirm. Too many affirmations can start to feel manipulative or fake. Choose your moments carefully and make them count.

Watch for affirmations that inadvertently carry expectations ("You're so strong, I know you can handle this"). While well-meaning, these can create pressure rather than support.

The Deeper Purpose

Affirmations do more than make people feel good. They help clients recognize resources they already possess for creating change. They build self-efficacy by highlighting past successes and current strengths. Most importantly, they help people see themselves as capable of positive change rather than as victims of their circumstances.

When you consistently notice and affirm genuine strengths, you help clients develop a more balanced and accurate self-perception. Instead of seeing only problems and deficits, they begin to recognize their own capabilities and positive qualities.

This shift in self-perception often becomes the foundation for lasting change. People who see themselves as resourceful, courageous, and capable are more likely to take the risks that change requires. They're also more likely to persist when efforts don't immediately succeed.

Chapter 7: Summary Statements - Pulling It Together Phrases

If reflections are the individual notes in a musical conversation, summaries are the chords that bring everything into harmony. They take the scattered pieces of what's been shared—the concerns, hopes, conflicts, and insights—and weave them into a coherent whole that both you and your client can understand.

Summaries serve multiple purposes in MI. They demonstrate that you've been tracking the big picture, not just individual moments. They help clients see patterns and connections they might have missed. Most importantly, they create natural transition points where conversations can shift direction or go deeper.

But summaries are more than just recaps. They're opportunities to highlight what's most important, amplify change talk, and help clients hear their own wisdom reflected back in an organized way. A well-crafted summary can help someone understand their situation more clearly and feel more confident about their next steps.

Collecting Summaries

These summaries gather together everything that's been shared during a conversation or session, organizing it in a way that makes sense of the whole.

Opening collecting summaries:

1. "Let me see if I understand what you've told me so far..."
2. "I want to make sure I'm following everything you've shared..."
3. "Let me pull together what I'm hearing from you..."

4. "So if I'm tracking with you correctly..."
5. "Here's what I'm understanding about your situation..."
6. "Let me see if I can capture the main themes of what you've been telling me..."
7. "I'd like to summarize what you've shared to make sure I understand..."

Structured collecting summaries:

8. "On one hand, you're feeling [X], but on the other hand, you're also experiencing [Y]."
9. "You've described several challenges: first [A], then [B], and also [C]."
10. "The main concerns you've raised are [X], [Y], and [Z]."
11. "You've talked about what's working: [positive elements], and also what's not working: [concerns]."
12. "There seem to be three main areas you're dealing with: your [relationship/work/health], your [second area], and your [third area]."

Research on therapeutic processes shows that periodic summarizing enhances client understanding and session effectiveness (Hill & Knox, 2009). These summaries help both counselor and client stay oriented to the bigger picture.

Linking Summaries

These summaries connect different pieces of information, helping clients see patterns or relationships they might not have recognized.

Pattern recognition summaries:

13. "I'm noticing a pattern where you [describe pattern] and then you feel [emotional consequence]."
14. "It seems like when [situation A] happens, you tend to [response], which leads to [outcome]."
15. "There's a connection between your [behavior/feeling] and your [value/goal] that comes up repeatedly."

16. "Each time you've talked about [topic], I hear [consistent theme]."
17. "The thread that runs through everything you've shared is [common element]."

Cause and effect summaries:

18. "When you try to [behavior], it seems to create [consequence], which then leads to [further result]."
19. "Your [positive intention] sometimes results in [unintended outcome]."
20. "The very thing that helps you [benefit] also creates [problem]."
21. "Your strength in [area] sometimes becomes a challenge when [situation]."

Change Talk Summaries

These summaries collect and amplify the client's own expressions of desire, ability, reasons, and need for change.

Desire and hope summaries:

22. "You've talked about wanting [specific changes] and hoping for [desired outcomes]."
23. "I hear how much you want things to be different, especially around [key areas]."
24. "Your vision for how you'd like things to be includes [elements of desired change]."
25. "You've expressed hoping for [specific hopes] and wanting to feel [desired emotions]."

Ability and confidence summaries:

26. "You've mentioned several strengths you have: [list specific strengths shared]."
27. "You've shown you can [past successes] and have the skills to [abilities mentioned]."

28. "From what you've told me, you have [resources] and the ability to [capabilities]."
29. "You've demonstrated that when you put your mind to something, you can [examples of past success]."

Reasons for change summaries:

30. "The reasons you've given for wanting change include [benefits they've mentioned]."
31. "You can see how [current situation] is affecting [important areas] and how change would [improve things]."
32. "The cost of staying the same includes [negative consequences], while changing could bring [benefits]."

Need and urgency summaries:

33. "You've said that something needs to change because [reasons for urgency]."
34. "There's a sense that you can't continue [current pattern] because [consequences]."
35. "You've reached a point where [situation] has become unacceptable."

Ambivalence Summaries

These summaries capture the natural conflicts and mixed feelings that most people experience when considering change.

Two-sided summaries:

36. "So you're torn between [one side] and [other side]."
37. "Part of you feels [one way] about this, while another part of you feels [different way]."
38. "You can see benefits to both [staying the same] and [changing]."
39. "There are things you'd gain by changing: [benefits], and things you might lose: [costs]."

40. "You have good reasons for [current behavior] and also good reasons for [changing behavior]."

Complex ambivalence summaries:

41. "This decision is complicated because [multiple factors]. You value [X] but you also need [Y], and you're concerned about [Z]."
42. "You want to [goal] because [reasons], but you're hesitant because [concerns], and you're also worried about [additional worries]."
43. "Your heart says [one thing], your head says [another thing], and the people around you are saying [third thing]."

Values and Meaning Summaries

These summaries help clients connect with what matters most to them and see how their concerns relate to their deeper values.

Values clarification summaries:

44. "What comes through clearly is how much you value [core values]."
45. "Being a good [parent/partner/employee] isn't just something you do—it's central to who you are."
46. "Your integrity matters more to you than your comfort."
47. "Family, authenticity, and [other values] are non-negotiable for you."
48. "You're willing to struggle for what matters rather than settle for what's easy."

Meaning-making summaries:

49. "This situation seems to be teaching you [lessons] about [insights]."
50. "You're not just dealing with [surface issue]—you're grappling with [deeper meaning]."
51. "This connects to bigger questions about [life themes]."

52. "What's really at stake here is [deeper meaning]."

Transition Summaries

These summaries help move conversations from one phase to another, often from exploration to action planning.

Shift to planning summaries:

53. "Given everything you've shared, what feels most important to focus on next?"
54. "So you've identified [problems] and [goals]—where would you like to start?"
55. "You've talked about several possible directions: [options]. Which one feels most right to you?"
56. "Now that we've explored [issues], what would you like to do with this information?"

Readiness summaries:

57. "You sound like someone who's ready to make some changes."
58. "There's an energy in your voice that suggests you're done just thinking about this."
59. "You've moved from wondering if you should change to figuring out how to change."
60. "Something has shifted for you—you're not just considering change anymore, you're planning for it."

Strength-Based Summaries

These summaries highlight the resources, skills, and positive qualities that clients bring to their change efforts.

Resource summaries:

61. "You have a lot of resources for dealing with this: [list resources mentioned]."

62. "Your support system includes [people], your skills include [abilities], and your experience includes [relevant past successes]."
63. "You're not starting from zero—you have [strengths] and [assets] to build on."

Character summaries:

64. "What comes through in everything you've shared is your [character traits]."
65. "Your [positive qualities] are evident in how you handle challenges."
66. "You're someone who [positive behavioral patterns] and cares deeply about [values]."

Closing Summaries

These summaries bring sessions to a close while reinforcing key insights or commitments.

Session wrap-up summaries:

67. "As we wrap up today, the main things we've covered are [key points]."
68. "Today you've [accomplishments in session] and identified [insights or goals]."
69. "We've talked about [main topics], and you've decided to [any commitments made]."
70. "The big picture from today is [overview of session content]."
71. "You came in with [initial concerns] and we've explored [what was discussed]."

Forward-looking summaries:

72. "Moving forward, you're planning to [intended actions] because [reasons]."

73. "Between now and next time, you want to [goals for interim period]."
74. "Your next steps include [planned actions] with the goal of [desired outcome]."
75. "You're taking away [insights] and planning to [intended changes]."

Crafting Effective Summaries

The best summaries are more than just recitations of what was said. They organize information in a way that makes sense, highlight what's most important, and often add perspective that helps clients understand their situations more clearly.

Start with the most important elements first. If someone has shared twelve different concerns, identify the two or three that seem most central and start there. You can always add other elements if needed.

Use the client's own language when possible. If they described feeling "stuck," use that word rather than substituting "trapped" or "immobilized." Their specific word choices often carry meaning that shouldn't be lost.

Pay attention to what you emphasize in summaries. Highlighting change talk and strengths tends to encourage more of the same. Focusing primarily on problems can inadvertently reinforce problem-focused thinking.

Getting Feedback on Summaries

Always check the accuracy of your summaries with clients. Use phrases like "Does that capture it?" or "What did I miss?" or "How does that sound to you?" Their corrections and additions often contain the most important information.

Some clients will say your summary is perfect when it's clearly incomplete. Others will correct minor details while missing major themes. Both responses give you useful information about how they process and organize information.

Don't take corrections as failures. When clients modify or correct your summaries, they're often clarifying their own thinking. The process of responding to your summary helps them understand their own experience better.

The Strategic Use of Summaries

Summaries can be powerful tools for guiding conversations without being directive. By choosing what to include and emphasize, you can highlight certain themes while downplaying others.

If a client has shared both change talk and sustain talk (reasons to stay the same), you might summarize by ending with the change talk: "So you're concerned about [problems] and you can see benefits to [current situation], and you're also feeling ready to [desired change]."

Summaries can also be used to introduce new perspectives or connections: "What I'm hearing is that your [behavior] might be your way of trying to [underlying positive intention], even though it's creating [unintended consequences]."

The Art of Strategic Incompleteness

Sometimes the most powerful summaries leave something out intentionally, inviting the client to complete the picture. You might summarize most of what they've shared but stop before the conclusion, letting them fill in the missing piece.

"So you've talked about how [situation] is affecting [areas of life], and you've mentioned that [circumstances], and you're feeling [emotions]..." Then pause and wait. Often clients will spontaneously add the insight or commitment you were hoping they'd reach.

This technique helps clients maintain ownership of their insights and decisions rather than feeling like you're leading them to predetermined conclusions.

These core responses—simple reflections, complex reflections, affirmations, and summaries—form the conversational backbone of Motivational Interviewing. Master these skills, and you'll have the tools to create the kind of therapeutic relationships where change becomes not just possible but inevitable.

But MI becomes even more powerful when you adapt these core skills to specific situations and populations. The next section explores how to use these foundational responses in the complex, messy realities of different counseling contexts. From substance abuse to health behaviors, from mental health to relationship issues, the same core principles apply—but the specific language and focus adapts to meet people exactly where they are.

Part III: Situation-Specific Scripts

The core MI responses you've learned form the foundation of every effective conversation about change. But real life doesn't happen in a vacuum. People come to you dealing with specific problems in particular contexts, each with its own language, concerns, and cultural dynamics.

A person struggling with alcohol use faces different challenges than someone managing diabetes or working through relationship conflicts. While the underlying MI principles remain the same, the specific words, concerns, and approaches need to adapt to each unique situation.

This section takes those core skills and shows you how to apply them in five common counseling contexts. You'll learn the specific language that works best for substance use issues, the particular concerns that arise in health behavior change, the unique challenges of mental health struggles, the complex dynamics of relationship problems, and the specific fears and hopes that accompany major life transitions.

Each situation requires you to understand not just the techniques but the lived experience of people facing these challenges. The scripts in these chapters aren't just different words—they're different ways of meeting people exactly where they are.

Chapter 8: Substance Use - Addiction-Specific Language

Talking about substance use requires a special kind of sensitivity. Most people who struggle with drugs or alcohol carry enormous shame about their relationship with substances. They've usually tried to quit or cut back multiple times. They've disappointed people they love. They may have done things while using that go against their values.

By the time someone sits across from you to discuss their substance use, they've likely heard plenty of lectures, ultimatums, and advice. They may be defensive, hopeless, or just going through the motions to satisfy someone else's requirements. Your job isn't to convince them they have a problem or tell them what they need to do. It's to help them explore their own relationship with substances and find their own motivation for change.

The language of addiction recovery has its own vocabulary, culture, and assumptions. Some clients embrace terms like "addict" or "alcoholic," while others find those labels stigmatizing or unhelpful. Some believe abstinence is the only solution, while others want to explore moderation. Your role is to meet people where they are, not where you think they should be.

Opening Conversations About Substance Use

Starting these conversations requires particular care. Many clients expect judgment, lectures, or demands for immediate change. Instead, you want to communicate curiosity and respect for their experience.

Non-judgmental openings:

1. "Tell me about your relationship with alcohol/drugs."
2. "How do substances fit into your life right now?"
3. "What's been your experience with drinking/using?"
4. "Help me understand the role that alcohol/drugs play for you."
5. "What's it like when you drink/use? What's it like when you don't?"
6. "How do you feel about your current pattern of substance use?"
7. "What concerns, if any, do you have about your drinking/drug use?"
8. "Other people have expressed concerns about your substance use. What are your thoughts about that?"

These openings avoid assumptions about whether someone has a "problem" and instead invite them to describe their own experience and perspective.

Exploring the Positive Functions

One of the biggest mistakes in addiction counseling is focusing only on the problems substances create while ignoring the benefits they provide. Most people use substances because they work—at least initially—to solve some problem or meet some need.

Exploring benefits:

9. "What does alcohol/drugs do for you that's helpful?"
10. "How do substances help you cope with things?"
11. "What would you miss most if you stopped using?"
12. "In what ways has drinking/using been a solution for you?"
13. "When you use, what changes for you that feels positive?"
14. "What needs do substances meet in your life?"
15. "How do drugs/alcohol help you handle stress?"
16. "What's working about your current pattern of use?"

Research consistently shows that exploring the positive functions of substance use reduces defensiveness and increases engagement (Miller & Rollnick, 2013). Clients often feel relieved when someone finally acknowledges that their substance use makes sense.

Reflecting Ambivalence

Most people with substance use issues feel torn between continuing to use and making changes. This ambivalence is normal and healthy—it means they're considering change. Your job is to help them explore both sides.

Two-sided reflections:

17. "Part of you enjoys drinking because it helps you relax, and part of you worries about how much you're consuming."
18. "You get something important from using, and you're also concerned about the impact on your health/relationships/work."
19. "On one hand, substances help you cope with stress, but on the other hand, they're creating new stresses."
20. "You want to cut back because of the problems it's causing, but you also don't want to give up something that helps you so much."
21. "You're torn between wanting to feel normal when you use and wanting to feel normal without using."

Exploring the costs:

22. "What concerns you about your current level of use?"
23. "How is drinking/using affecting things that matter to you?"
24. "What problems has substance use created in your life?"
25. "What are you losing because of your relationship with alcohol/drugs?"
26. "How is your use impacting your relationships/work/health/goals?"
27. "What would be different in your life if substances weren't part of the picture?"

Language Around Control and Choice

Many people struggling with substances feel like their use is out of control. Others maintain they can stop anytime. Both perspectives need to be explored without judgment.

Exploring control:

28. "How much control do you feel you have over your drinking/using?"
29. "What's it like when you try to cut back or stop?"
30. "Tell me about times when you've been able to moderate or abstain."
31. "When do you feel most in control of your use? When do you feel least in control?"
32. "How do you decide when, where, and how much to use?"
33. "What makes the difference between using as planned and using more than you intended?"

Reflecting loss of control:

34. "Sometimes your use goes according to plan, and sometimes it surprises you."
35. "You start with good intentions, but substances can have their own agenda."
36. "There's a part of you that makes decisions about using, and a part that seems to take over once you start."
37. "You want to be in the driver's seat, but sometimes substances seem to be driving."

Exploring Identity and Labels

The language people use to describe themselves matters enormously. Some embrace recovery terminology, others reject it entirely. Your job is to understand their perspective, not impose your own.

Exploring self-perception:

38. "How do you see yourself in relation to your substance use?"
39. "What words would you use to describe your relationship with alcohol/drugs?"
40. "How do you feel about terms like 'addict' or 'alcoholic'? Do they fit for you?"
41. "Some people identify as having an addiction, others see it differently. What feels true for you?"
42. "How has your identity changed as your relationship with substances has changed?"

Avoiding labels while staying supportive:

43. "Whatever you want to call it, you're dealing with something that's causing problems."
44. "Labels matter less than your experience and what you want to do about it."
45. "The words don't matter as much as how you're feeling and what you want for yourself."
46. "You get to decide how you understand your relationship with substances."

Discussing Previous Change Efforts

Most people have tried to quit or cut back before. These previous efforts often feel like failures, but they're actually valuable learning experiences.

Exploring past attempts:

47. "Tell me about times you've tried to change your drinking/using."
48. "What approaches have you tried before? How did they work?"
49. "What was most helpful during times when you were able to cut back or stop?"
50. "What made the difference between successful periods and times when you went back to using?"

51. "What did you learn about yourself from previous attempts to change?"
52. "What worked for a while, even if it didn't work long-term?"

Reframing "relapses":

53. "What you're calling failure sounds like learning to me."
54. "Every attempt teaches you something about what works and what doesn't."
55. "You haven't failed—you've gathered information about what you need to succeed."
56. "Each time you try, you're building skills and understanding."
57. "Going back to using doesn't erase the progress you made."

Research on the stages of change shows that most people cycle through multiple attempts before achieving sustained change (Prochaska & DiClemente, 1983). Reframing previous attempts as learning experiences reduces shame and maintains hope.

Addressing Family and Relationship Impact

Substance use rarely affects only the person using. Family members, friends, and coworkers are often impacted, and their responses can either support or complicate recovery efforts.

Exploring relationship impact:

58. "How is your use affecting people you care about?"
59. "What do the important people in your life say about your drinking/using?"
60. "How do you feel about the impact your substance use has on your family/partner/children?"
61. "What would your loved ones say if they knew you were considering changing?"
62. "How would your relationships be different if substances weren't part of the picture?"

When family is pressuring change:

63. "It sounds like other people want you to change more than you do right now."
64. "How do you feel about making changes because others want you to versus making changes because you want to?"
65. "What's it like to have people monitoring your use and pressuring you to quit?"
66. "You might change for yourself at some point, even if you're not ready to change for others right now."
67. "Being pushed to change can sometimes make us want to resist, even when part of us agrees with the concern."

Exploring Goals and Options

Not everyone needs or wants complete abstinence. While some situations require sobriety, others allow for exploration of moderation. Your job is to help clients think through their options realistically.

Exploring change goals:

68. "What changes, if any, would you like to make regarding your substance use?"
69. "If you decided to change your relationship with alcohol/drugs, what would that look like?"
70. "Some people aim for complete abstinence, others work on moderation. What makes sense for you?"
71. "What would success look like for you when it comes to your substance use?"
72. "How would you know if you were in a healthier relationship with substances?"

Moderation versus abstinence:

73. "Tell me about your thoughts on moderating versus stopping completely."

74. "What appeals to you about the idea of controlled use? What concerns you about it?"
75. "Some substances and some people work better with moderation, others with abstinence. What fits for your situation?"
76. "What would need to be different for moderation to work for you?"

When abstinence seems necessary:

77. "Given what you've told me about your attempts to moderate, what do you make of that?"
78. "Some people find that complete abstinence is actually easier than trying to control their use."
79. "You've tried moderation several times without success. What does that tell you?"
80. "For some people and some substances, an on/off switch works better than a dimmer switch."

Discussing Treatment and Support Options

Many clients have preconceptions about addiction treatment that might prevent them from considering helpful options. Your role is to provide accurate information without pressuring specific choices.

Exploring treatment options:

81. "What are your thoughts about getting additional support for changing your substance use?"
82. "What's your understanding of what treatment involves?"
83. "Have you ever considered counseling, groups, or other forms of support?"
84. "What would make you more open to seeking additional help?"
85. "What would treatment need to look like for it to be appealing to you?"

Addressing treatment resistance:

86. "It sounds like you have some concerns about formal treatment."
87. "What would you need to know about treatment options to feel more comfortable?"
88. "Not all treatment is the same. What approach would fit best with your personality and situation?"
89. "You don't have to do this alone, but you get to choose what kind of support makes sense."
90. "What's worked for other people might not work for you, and what works for you might be different from what worked for others."

Handling Setbacks and Slips

When clients return to substance use after a period of abstinence or reduced use, they often feel ashamed and hopeless. Your response in these moments can determine whether they give up or keep trying.

Responding to slips:

91. "What happened that led you back to using?"
92. "You used again, and you're here talking about it. That tells me you haven't given up."
93. "What did you learn about yourself or your triggers from this experience?"
94. "Slips often teach us something important about what we need to do differently."
95. "You had [length of time] of success before this happened. That shows you can do it."
96. "What would you do differently if you found yourself in that same situation again?"

Maintaining hope after setbacks:

97. "This doesn't erase all the progress you've made."
98. "Many people need multiple attempts before they find what works."
99. "You're learning what your recovery needs to look like."

100.　　　"The fact that you're disappointed about using shows how much change matters to you."

Working with Denial and Minimization

Some clients genuinely don't see their substance use as problematic. Others minimize the extent of problems to protect themselves from painful realizations or unwanted pressure to change.

Responding to denial:

101.　　　"You don't see your use as a problem, but others in your life do. What do you make of that difference in perspective?"
102.　　　"Help me understand why you think your drinking/using is fine while others are concerned."
103.　　　"What would have to happen for you to think your substance use was becoming a problem?"
104.　　　"You and [family member/employer/court] seem to see this situation very differently."

When minimizing consequences:

105.　　　"Those problems might seem small to you, but they brought you here."
106.　　　"Even if the consequences seem minor now, they might be pointing toward bigger concerns."
107.　　　"You're handling the problems that have come up so far, but what if they got worse?"
108.　　　"Some people find that problems with substances tend to grow over time, not stay the same."

Special Considerations for Different Substances

Different substances create different patterns of use and different types of problems. Your language should adapt to the specific substance and its effects.

For alcohol:

109. "Drinking is so common in our culture that it can be hard to know when it crosses a line."
110. "You can buy alcohol anywhere and use it legally, which makes it different from other drugs."
111. "Most people drink without problems, so it makes sense that you'd wonder if yours is really an issue."

For prescription medications:

112. "These medications were prescribed for legitimate medical reasons, which makes this situation complex."
113. "The line between medical use and misuse isn't always clear."
114. "You started taking these for real health problems, and now you're dealing with unexpected complications."

For illegal substances:

115. "Using illegal drugs adds legal risks on top of the health and personal risks."
116. "The illegality makes it harder to get help or talk openly about problems."
117. "You're dealing with substance issues plus the stress of doing something illegal."

The Marathon, Not the Sprint

Working with substance use issues requires patience and realistic expectations. Change is usually a process, not an event. People often need multiple attempts and different approaches before finding what works.

Your role is to plant seeds, provide support, and maintain hope even when clients aren't ready to make changes. Sometimes the most important thing you do is help someone feel less alone with their struggle and more hopeful about the possibility of change.

The language you use matters enormously. Words that convey respect, curiosity, and hope can open doors that have been slammed shut by shame, stigma, and previous negative experiences with helping professionals. When you speak to the whole person rather than just the problem, you create space for healing and growth that goes far beyond just stopping substance use.

Chapter 9: Health Behaviors - Medical and Lifestyle Phrases

Health behavior change sits at a unique intersection. It's deeply personal but often involves medical professionals. It requires lifestyle changes that affect daily routines, family dynamics, and social relationships. Most challenging of all, it usually involves changing habits that are automatic, pleasurable, or help people cope with stress.

Whether someone needs to manage diabetes, lose weight, exercise more, quit smoking, or follow a medication regimen, they're facing the same basic challenge: changing patterns that are woven into the fabric of their daily life. Unlike other types of problems that might be addressed once and resolved, health behaviors require ongoing attention and consistent choices.

The scripts in this chapter acknowledge the unique challenges of health behavior change while respecting the reality that people are experts on their own bodies and lives. They help clients explore their own motivations for change while working within medical realities and recommendations.

Starting Health Behavior Conversations

Many clients come to health behavior discussions with anxiety, shame, or resignation. They may have tried multiple times to make changes. They might be dealing with scary diagnoses or pressure from medical providers. Your opening sets the tone for whether this will be another lecture or a collaborative exploration.

Non-judgmental health openings:

1. "How are you feeling about the health changes your doctor recommended?"
2. "What's it been like for you to hear about [diagnosis/health concern]?"
3. "Tell me about your thoughts on making these lifestyle changes."
4. "How do you see your health situation right now?"
5. "What concerns you most about your current health?"
6. "What questions do you have about what your doctor told you?"
7. "How are you handling the idea of needing to make some changes?"
8. "What's been on your mind since your medical appointment?"

These openings invite clients to share their perspective rather than assuming they're motivated to change or understand what they need to do.

Exploring Current Health Behaviors

Before discussing changes, it's important to understand current patterns without judgment. Many clients expect criticism, so your curiosity about their current approach can be disarming.

Understanding current patterns:

9. "Walk me through a typical day in terms of eating/exercise/medication."
10. "What does your current routine look like when it comes to [health behavior]?"
11. "How do you currently manage your [condition/symptoms]?"
12. "What's working well about how you're taking care of yourself now?"
13. "Tell me about the health habits you already have in place."
14. "What have you tried before when it comes to [health behavior]?"

15. "How do you fit health-related activities into your current schedule?"
16. "What makes it easier or harder to take care of your health?"

Acknowledging the Difficulty of Health Changes

Health behavior change is genuinely difficult. Acknowledging this reality validates clients' experiences and reduces shame about previous "failures."

Validating difficulty:

17. "Changing eating habits is one of the hardest things people do."
18. "Exercise is challenging to fit into an already busy life."
19. "Taking medications consistently is harder than most people realize."
20. "Managing a chronic condition requires constant attention and decision-making."
21. "Your body is used to the way you've been living, so change feels uncomfortable."
22. "You're being asked to change habits you've had for years or decades."
23. "Health changes affect not just you but your whole family's routines."
24. "It's frustrating when you know what you should do but doing it feels overwhelming."

Research shows that acknowledging the difficulty of behavior change increases rather than decreases motivation (Rollnick et al., 2008). When clients feel understood, they're more likely to engage honestly in problem-solving.

Exploring Personal Motivation

Medical recommendations provide the "what" of health behavior change, but personal motivation provides the "why." Your job is to help clients connect with their own reasons for wanting to be healthier.

Finding personal reasons:

25. "What would you gain by making these health changes?"
26. "How would improving your health affect the things that matter most to you?"
27. "What would be different in your daily life if you felt healthier?"
28. "Who in your life would be affected if your health improved?"
29. "What activities would you be able to do if you felt better physically?"
30. "How would taking better care of yourself change how you feel about yourself?"
31. "What's your biggest fear about what might happen if your health gets worse?"

Connecting to values:

32. "Being around for your grandchildren seems really important to you."
33. "You want to be a good example for your kids when it comes to healthy living."
34. "Having energy for work and family matters to you."
35. "Independence and not being a burden on others is a core value for you."
36. "You take pride in taking care of yourself."
37. "Quality of life matters more to you than just living longer."

Working with Medical Anxiety and Fear

Health concerns often bring up fears about mortality, disability, or loss of independence. These fears can either motivate change or create paralyzing anxiety.

Addressing health anxiety:

38. "It sounds scary to think about what might happen if you don't make changes."
39. "Learning about your diagnosis has brought up a lot of worries."
40. "The uncertainty about your health future is really difficult."
41. "You're dealing with fear on top of trying to change your habits."
42. "It's hard to know how much to worry and how much to stay hopeful."
43. "The medical information you've received feels overwhelming."

Balancing hope and realism:

44. "You want to be realistic about your health without losing hope."
45. "Taking action gives you some control over things that feel out of control."
46. "Making changes can't guarantee outcomes, but it can improve your odds."
47. "You're doing what you can do and accepting what you can't control."

Addressing All-or-Nothing Thinking

Many clients approach health changes with perfectionist attitudes that set them up for failure. Helping them think in terms of progress rather than perfection is crucial.

Encouraging moderation:

48. "You don't have to be perfect to make a real difference in your health."
49. "Small, consistent changes often work better than dramatic overhauls."
50. "Progress matters more than perfection."
51. "Every healthy choice you make counts, even if you make unhealthy choices too."
52. "You can improve your health significantly without completely changing your lifestyle."
53. "It's better to make changes you can sustain than changes that are dramatic but temporary."

When clients have "blown it":

54. "One bad day doesn't cancel out all the good days."
55. "You can get back on track without starting completely over."
56. "What matters is your overall pattern, not individual choices."
57. "You're learning what works and what doesn't. This information is valuable."

Working with Family and Social Challenges

Health behavior changes affect entire family systems and social relationships. Spouses might resist dietary changes, friends might not understand exercise priorities, or family members might sabotage efforts unconsciously.

Addressing social challenges:

58. "How is your family responding to the changes you're trying to make?"
59. "What's it like to eat differently from the people you live with?"
60. "How do social situations affect your ability to stick with your health goals?"

61. "Who in your life supports your health changes? Who makes it more difficult?"
62. "How do you handle it when others pressure you to make unhealthy choices?"
63. "What would help your family understand and support what you're trying to do?"

When family undermines efforts:

64. "It's hard to make changes when the people closest to you aren't on board."
65. "You're trying to take care of your health while also maintaining your relationships."
66. "Sometimes people resist our changes because they're afraid of how it will affect them."
67. "You might need to make changes for yourself even if others don't understand or support them."

Medication Adherence

Taking medications consistently is a common challenge that involves more than just memory. Issues include side effects, cost, complexity of regimens, and beliefs about medication.

Exploring medication concerns:

68. "What's your experience been like taking these medications?"
69. "How do you feel about having to take medication long-term?"
70. "What makes it easy or difficult to remember to take your medications?"
71. "How do the side effects affect your daily life?"
72. "What concerns do you have about taking these medications?"
73. "How does the cost of medications affect your ability to take them consistently?"

74. "What would make it easier to stick with your medication routine?"

When clients resist medication:

75. "You have mixed feelings about taking medication for this condition."
76. "It's hard to take medications when you feel fine without them."
77. "You're weighing the benefits of medication against the downsides."
78. "Taking medication makes the condition feel more real and permanent."
79. "You'd rather manage your condition without medication if possible."

Diet and Nutrition Changes

Food is deeply connected to culture, family, emotions, and social relationships. Dietary changes can feel like losses of identity, pleasure, or connection with others.

Discussing food changes:

80. "Food means more than just nutrition in your life."
81. "Changing how you eat affects social situations and family traditions."
82. "You're being asked to give up foods that bring you comfort or joy."
83. "Eating healthier costs more money and takes more time to prepare."
84. "You want to eat well, but you also want to enjoy your food."
85. "The foods you're supposed to avoid are the ones you enjoy most."

When clients feel deprived:

86. "This feels like you're losing things you enjoy rather than gaining health."
87. "It's hard to feel motivated about changes that feel like punishment."
88. "You want to find a way to eat healthily that doesn't feel like constant sacrifice."
89. "Food restrictions make you feel different from everyone else."

Exercise and Physical Activity

Exercise recommendations often clash with reality for people dealing with time constraints, physical limitations, financial issues, or past negative experiences with physical activity.

Discussing exercise barriers:

90. "Finding time to exercise in an already packed schedule is challenging."
91. "Your body feels different now than it did when you were younger."
92. "Past injuries or pain make exercise feel risky."
93. "You've never enjoyed traditional forms of exercise."
94. "Gyms and fitness centers don't feel comfortable or welcoming to you."
95. "You're embarrassed about your current fitness level."

Finding acceptable activities:

96. "What types of physical activity have you enjoyed in the past?"
97. "Exercise doesn't have to mean going to a gym or running."
98. "What would make moving your body feel good rather than like work?"
99. "How could you add more activity to things you already do?"
100. "What would need to be different for exercise to feel doable?"

Weight Management

Weight loss is one of the most common health behavior changes, and it's loaded with shame, previous failures, and societal judgment. Clients need support that acknowledges the complexity beyond "eat less, move more."

Sensitive weight discussions:

101.   "Your relationship with your weight has been complicated."
102.   "You've tried to lose weight many times, and it's been frustrating."
103.   "Weight is affected by many factors, some of which are outside your control."
104.   "You want to be healthier, and you're not sure if that requires losing weight."
105.   "Society gives a lot of messages about weight that don't match your experience."
106.   "You're tired of your weight being the focus when there are other health issues that matter too."

When focusing on behaviors rather than weight:

107.   "What if we focused on healthy behaviors rather than the number on the scale?"
108.   "Your body will find its natural weight when you consistently take care of it."
109.   "Health improvements might happen before weight changes."
110.   "You can be healthier at your current weight by changing some behaviors."

Chronic Disease Management

Living with conditions like diabetes, heart disease, or autoimmune disorders requires ongoing attention and lifestyle adjustments. The psychological impact often gets overlooked.

Acknowledging chronic illness challenges:

111. "Managing this condition requires constant decisions and attention."
112. "Your whole life has changed since your diagnosis."
113. "It's exhausting to have to think about your health all the time."
114. "You're grieving the loss of your previous relationship with your body."
115. "This condition affects not just your physical health but your emotional well-being."
116. "You're learning to live with uncertainty about your health future."

Supporting self-management:

117. "You're becoming an expert on your own condition and body."
118. "You know better than anyone how this condition affects you personally."
119. "You're developing skills to manage something that's genuinely difficult."
120. "Taking care of a chronic condition is a full-time job on top of everything else you do."

Working with Setbacks

Health behavior change is rarely linear. Clients will have good days and bad days, periods of success and periods of struggle. How you handle setbacks often determines whether clients give up or keep trying.

Responding to health behavior slips:

121. "You had a rough week with your eating/exercise/medication routine."
122. "What happened that made it harder to stick with your health goals?"

123.   "You're disappointed about the choices you made, and you're here talking about getting back on track."
124.   "Setbacks are part of the process for most people making health changes."
125.   "What did you learn about yourself or your triggers from this experience?"

Maintaining momentum after setbacks:

126.   "You had [length of time] of success before this rough patch."
127.   "The progress you made before didn't disappear because you had some difficult days."
128.   "What worked before can work again."
129.   "You know more now about what you need to succeed than you did when you started."
130.   "Every time you get back on track, you're building resilience and problem-solving skills."

The Integration Challenge

Health behavior change isn't just about learning new habits—it's about integrating those habits into a life that's already full and complex. Your role is to help clients find ways to be healthier that fit with their real lives, not some idealized version of how they think they should live.

The most effective health behavior changes are ones that clients choose based on their own values and priorities, implemented in ways that work with their schedules, resources, and relationships. When you help people connect with their own motivation and adapt recommendations to their real lives, you increase the chances that changes will be sustainable rather than temporary.

Chapter 10: Mental Health - Depression, Anxiety, Trauma Responses

Mental health struggles create their own unique language and challenges. Unlike substance use or health behaviors that involve specific actions to change, mental health issues often feel internal, pervasive, and beyond voluntary control. Someone dealing with depression might say "I am depressed" rather than "I do depressed things," highlighting how mental health conditions can become part of identity in ways that complicate change efforts.

The symptoms themselves create barriers to change. Depression saps motivation and energy. Anxiety creates avoidance and catastrophic thinking. Trauma responses can make it difficult to trust others or feel safe enough to be vulnerable. These conditions often involve negative thought patterns that have been reinforced for years or decades.

Your role isn't to talk someone out of their depression or convince them their anxiety is irrational. Instead, you want to help them explore their relationship with their symptoms, find their own motivations for feeling different, and discover their existing strengths and resources for managing mental health challenges.

Opening Mental Health Conversations

Many clients come to mental health discussions carrying shame, hopelessness, or fear about their symptoms. They might worry about being seen as "crazy," weak, or broken. Your opening needs to communicate safety and normalize their experience.

Safe mental health openings:

1. "How are you doing with everything that's been going on?"
2. "What brings you here today? What's been on your mind?"
3. "Tell me about how you've been feeling lately."
4. "What's it been like for you to be struggling with [depression/anxiety/trauma responses]?"
5. "How has your mental health been affecting your daily life?"
6. "What's the hardest part about what you're experiencing right now?"
7. "How long have you been dealing with these feelings?"
8. "What made you decide to seek help at this point?"

These openings invite clients to describe their experience without pathologizing or minimizing their symptoms.

Exploring the Impact of Symptoms

Mental health symptoms ripple through every aspect of life. Helping clients articulate this impact can increase motivation for change while validating their struggles.

Understanding symptom impact:

9. "How is depression/anxiety affecting your relationships?"
10. "What's different about your life now compared to when you were feeling better?"
11. "How are these symptoms interfering with things that matter to you?"
12. "What have you had to give up or change because of how you're feeling?"
13. "How is your mental health affecting your work/school performance?"
14. "What's it like to try to function normally when you're feeling this way inside?"
15. "How do you explain to others what you're going through?"
16. "What's been the most frustrating part of dealing with these symptoms?"

Research shows that helping clients connect symptoms to functional impairment increases motivation for treatment engagement (Kazdin, 2007). These questions help clients see the full scope of how mental health affects their lives.

Addressing Hopelessness and Despair

Hopelessness is often a central feature of mental health struggles. Clients may feel like they'll never get better, that nothing will help, or that they're fundamentally damaged. This hopelessness needs to be acknowledged without being reinforced.

Responding to hopelessness:

17. "You've been suffering for so long that it's hard to imagine feeling different."
18. "Right now it feels like this is just how you are, not something that can change."
19. "You've tried things before that didn't help, so it makes sense you'd feel discouraged."
20. "The depression/anxiety is telling you that nothing will work, but that's what these conditions do."
21. "It's hard to have hope when you're in the middle of feeling so bad."
22. "You can't see the light at the end of the tunnel right now."

Gentle hope building:

23. "Even small improvements would make a difference in how you feel."
24. "You don't have to feel great to feel better than you do now."
25. "Mental health conditions are treatable, even when they don't feel like it."
26. "You've gotten through difficult periods before."
27. "The fact that you're here suggests part of you still believes change is possible."
28. "Hope doesn't have to feel strong to be real."

Working with Depression

Depression creates a specific set of challenges including low energy, negative thinking patterns, loss of interest in activities, and feelings of worthlessness. The symptoms themselves make it hard to engage in activities that might help.

Understanding depression:

29. "It takes enormous energy just to get through basic daily tasks."
30. "Nothing feels enjoyable or rewarding the way it used to."
31. "Your brain is telling you negative things about yourself and your future."
32. "You feel disconnected from people even when they're trying to help."
33. "Everything feels harder and takes more effort than it should."
34. "You're dealing with both feeling bad and feeling bad about feeling bad."

Depression-specific motivational responses:

35. "Even though you don't feel like doing anything, you're here talking about change."
36. "You're fighting against your brain's messages that nothing will help."
37. "Getting out of bed and coming here took real courage when you feel this way."
38. "You care about your family even though depression makes it hard to show it."
39. "Part of you remembers what it was like to feel better."
40. "You want to be present for your life even when everything feels gray."

Working with Anxiety

Anxiety creates avoidance patterns, catastrophic thinking, and physical symptoms that can feel overwhelming. Clients often feel like they should be able to "just relax" but can't control their worried thoughts or physical reactions.

Understanding anxiety:

41. "Your mind goes to worst-case scenarios automatically."
42. "The physical symptoms of anxiety feel scary and real."
43. "You avoid situations that might trigger anxiety, which limits your life."
44. "You're exhausted from being on high alert all the time."
45. "Other people don't understand how difficult everyday situations can be for you."
46. "You want to feel calm, but your brain and body have different ideas."

Anxiety-specific motivational responses:

47. "You keep pushing yourself to do things despite feeling anxious."
48. "You're brave enough to face situations that genuinely feel scary to you."
49. "You want to expand your world instead of letting anxiety make it smaller."
50. "You're tired of anxiety making decisions for you."
51. "You know logically that most of your worries don't come true, but knowing that doesn't make them feel less real."
52. "You want to trust yourself to handle whatever comes up."

Working with Trauma Responses

Trauma creates complex responses including hypervigilance, emotional numbing, intrusive memories, and difficulty trusting others. Clients may feel like they're fundamentally changed by their experiences.

Understanding trauma impacts:

53. "Your brain and body are still reacting to danger even when you're safe."
54. "Trust feels risky when you've been hurt before."
55. "Parts of you feel stuck in the past while other parts are trying to move forward."
56. "You're protecting yourself in ways that made sense then but might not fit your life now."
57. "Your reactions are normal responses to abnormal experiences."
58. "You're dealing with both the original trauma and how it continues to affect you."

Trauma-informed motivational responses:

59. "You survived something terrible, which shows incredible strength."
60. "You're here seeking help despite how hard it is to trust."
61. "You want to reclaim parts of yourself that trauma took away."
62. "You're tired of the past controlling your present."
63. "You deserve to feel safe and peaceful in your own body."
64. "Healing doesn't mean forgetting—it means the memories don't control you."

Exploring Coping Strategies

Most clients have developed some ways of managing their mental health symptoms. Some strategies are helpful, others are problematic, and many are mixed. Understanding current coping helps you build on strengths.

Understanding current coping:

65. "How do you get through the really difficult days?"
66. "What helps you feel even slightly better when symptoms are bad?"

67. "What strategies have you tried for managing your mental health?"
68. "Who or what do you turn to for support when you're struggling?"
69. "What gets you out of bed on the days when you don't want to?"
70. "How do you take care of yourself when symptoms flare up?"

Problematic coping responses:

71. "Some of your coping strategies help in the short term but might be costly long term."
72. "You've found ways to numb the pain, but they also numb everything else."
73. "The behaviors that help you feel safe might also be keeping you isolated."
74. "You're doing what you need to do to survive, even if it's not ideal."

Addressing Shame and Self-Criticism

Mental health struggles often involve harsh self-judgment. Clients may feel weak, broken, or defective. This shame can be more painful than the original symptoms and creates barriers to seeking help and making changes.

Responding to shame:

75. "Mental health conditions are not character flaws or personal weaknesses."
76. "You didn't choose to feel this way, and it's not your fault."
77. "Having a mental health condition doesn't make you less valuable as a person."
78. "You're being harder on yourself than you would be on anyone else with the same struggles."
79. "The voice in your head that says you're broken is part of the problem, not the truth about who you are."

80. "You deserve compassion, especially from yourself."

Challenging self-critical thoughts:

81. "What would you tell a friend who was going through exactly what you're experiencing?"
82. "You're treating yourself like an enemy when you need to be your own ally."
83. "That critical voice might think it's helping, but it's actually making things worse."
84. "You can acknowledge your struggles without defining yourself by them."

Working with Identity and Mental Health

Mental health conditions can become so pervasive that people begin to see them as core parts of their identity. This can create resistance to change because getting better might feel like losing part of themselves.

Exploring identity issues:

85. "You've been dealing with this for so long that it feels like part of who you are."
86. "It's scary to think about changing when this has been your normal for so long."
87. "You might not remember what you were like before these symptoms started."
88. "Part of you wonders if you'd still be you without the depression/anxiety."
89. "These conditions have shaped how you see yourself and how others see you."

Separating person from symptoms:

90. "You are not your depression/anxiety/trauma—you're a person dealing with these conditions."

91. "Your mental health symptoms are something you have, not something you are."
92. "You existed before these symptoms, and you'll exist after they improve."
93. "The real you is still there underneath the symptoms."

Discussing Treatment Options

Many clients have preconceptions about mental health treatment based on stigma, previous experiences, or media portrayals. Your job is to provide accurate information while respecting their autonomy.

Exploring treatment attitudes:

94. "What are your thoughts about therapy/medication/other treatments?"
95. "What has your experience been with mental health professionals in the past?"
96. "What would make you more open to trying treatment?"
97. "What concerns do you have about getting help for your mental health?"
98. "What would treatment need to look like for it to feel right for you?"

When clients resist treatment:

99. "You're not sure that therapy/medication would actually help."
100. "You've managed on your own this long, so seeking help feels like admitting defeat."
101. "You're worried about side effects or becoming dependent on treatment."
102. "Part of you wants help, and part of you is skeptical that anything will work."
103. "You don't want to be seen as crazy or damaged by getting professional help."

Medication Conversations

Psychiatric medications often bring up complex feelings about identity, dependence, and stigma. Some clients see medication as a sign of weakness, while others see it as essential for functioning.

Exploring medication attitudes:

104.   "How do you feel about the possibility of taking medication for your mental health?"
105.   "What concerns do you have about psychiatric medications?"
106.   "What would it mean to you to need medication to feel normal?"
107.   "How do you balance the potential benefits and risks of medication?"
108.   "What questions do you have about how these medications work?"

When clients resist medication:

109.   "You'd rather handle this without medication if possible."
110.   "Taking psychiatric medication feels like giving up or admitting something's wrong with you."
111.   "You're worried about side effects or becoming dependent."
112.   "You want to be yourself, not a medicated version of yourself."

When clients want medication:

113.   "You're ready to try anything that might help you feel better."
114.   "Medication feels like hope when nothing else has worked."
115.   "You see medication as a tool, not a sign of weakness."

Building on Existing Strengths

Even in the midst of mental health struggles, clients possess resources and strengths. Identifying these can provide foundation for change and counter negative self-perceptions.

Identifying mental health strengths:

116. "You've survived every difficult day so far, which shows remarkable resilience."
117. "You're seeking help, which takes courage when you're feeling vulnerable."
118. "You care about how your mental health affects others, which shows your compassion."
119. "You keep trying even when previous attempts haven't worked."
120. "You're able to recognize when you're struggling, which is an important skill."
121. "You have insights into your patterns and triggers."
122. "You've maintained some functioning even while dealing with these symptoms."

The Complexity of Mental Health Change

Mental health recovery isn't linear or simple. Good days and bad days can alternate unpredictably. Symptoms might improve in some areas while remaining problematic in others. Progress often feels slow and sometimes invisible.

Your role is to help clients maintain hope during the difficult periods, celebrate small improvements, and remember that recovery is possible even when it doesn't feel that way. The language you use can either reinforce negative self-perceptions or help clients see themselves as capable of healing and growth.

Most importantly, you want to help clients reclaim agency in their lives. Mental health conditions can make people feel powerless and out of control. When you help them identify choices they can make and strengths they possess, you're supporting their movement from victim to survivor to thriver.

Chapter 11: Relationship Issues - Couples and Family Dynamics

Relationship problems create a unique set of challenges for MI practitioners. Unlike individual issues where you're helping one person explore their motivation for change, relationship work involves multiple people with different perspectives, needs, and goals. Each person usually sees the other as the one who needs to change, while minimizing their own contributions to problems.

The dynamics that create relationship problems—blame, defensiveness, criticism, contempt—are the same dynamics that can emerge in couples counseling if you're not careful. Your job is to create safety for honest communication while helping each person explore their own role in both the problems and the solutions.

MI principles translate beautifully to relationship work, but they require adaptation. You'll need to reflect multiple perspectives simultaneously, affirm each person's experience while not taking sides, and help couples find shared motivations for change while respecting individual autonomy.

Opening Relationship Conversations

When couples or families come to counseling, tension is often high. People may be angry, hurt, or defensive. Your opening needs to create safety for everyone while acknowledging that there are multiple valid perspectives in the room.

Safe relationship openings:

1. "What brings you both here today? What are you hoping we can work on together?"

2. "How would each of you describe what's been happening in your relationship?"
3. "What made you decide to seek counseling at this point?"
4. "I'd like to hear from both of you about how you see the situation."
5. "What are your biggest concerns about your relationship right now?"
6. "Tell me what's been most difficult about your relationship lately."
7. "What would you each like to see change in your relationship?"
8. "How are you both feeling about being here today?"

These openings invite multiple perspectives without assuming who's at fault or what needs to change.

Managing Blame and Criticism

Most couples arrive with a list of complaints about their partner. While these concerns may be valid, blame and criticism shut down productive conversation. Your job is to acknowledge concerns while redirecting toward personal responsibility.

Responding to blame:

9. "You're really frustrated with how [partner] handles [situation]."
10. "It sounds like you feel hurt by [specific behavior] and want that to change."
11. "You're feeling unheard when [partner] does [behavior]."
12. "Your needs aren't being met in this area, and that's painful."
13. "You'd like [partner] to understand how their actions affect you."
14. "You care so much about this relationship that these issues feel urgent."

Redirecting from blame to personal experience:

15. "Instead of focusing on what [partner] does wrong, tell me what you need to feel loved/safe/valued."
16. "What would you like to be different about how you handle conflict together?"
17. "How do you typically respond when [situation] happens?"
18. "What role do you play in the patterns you're concerned about?"
19. "What could you do differently that might change the dynamic?"

Research shows that taking personal responsibility for relationship problems, rather than blaming partners, predicts better treatment outcomes (Jacobson & Addis, 1993). These responses help shift from accusation to exploration.

Exploring Each Person's Perspective

In relationship work, everyone needs to feel heard and understood. This means reflecting each person's experience without agreeing or disagreeing with their interpretation.

Validating multiple perspectives:

20. "From your perspective, [summarize their view]. And from your perspective, [summarize partner's view]."
21. "You each have different experiences of the same events."
22. "Both of your feelings make sense given how you're experiencing the situation."
23. "You're both hurting, just in different ways."
24. "Each of you is trying to get needs met, but in ways that don't work for the other person."
25. "Your intentions are good, but the impact on each other is problematic."

When perspectives conflict:

26. "You remember this situation very differently from each other."

27. "The same event affected each of you in different ways."
28. "You're both telling the truth about your experience, even though the stories don't match."
29. "Facts matter less than how each of you felt during these interactions."
30. "Your different perspectives help explain why this has been so confusing."

Identifying Underlying Needs

Most relationship conflicts are about surface issues that represent deeper needs. Helping couples identify underlying needs creates possibilities for solutions that work for everyone.

Exploring deeper needs:

31. "When [partner] does [behavior], what do you need that you're not getting?"
32. "What would help you feel more loved/respected/safe in this relationship?"
33. "What do you miss most from earlier in your relationship?"
34. "What would need to happen for you to feel more connected to each other?"
35. "What are you afraid would happen if things don't improve?"
36. "What do you need from [partner] to feel like a team again?"

Common relationship needs:

37. "You need to feel heard and understood, not just tolerated."
38. "Feeling appreciated and valued is important to you."
39. "You want to feel like you matter and your feelings count."
40. "Safety—emotional and physical—is essential for you."
41. "You need to feel like you're partners, not adversaries."
42. "Intimacy and connection are priorities for you."

Working with Communication Patterns

Most couples have developed negative communication patterns that reinforce problems. These patterns often feel automatic and can be changed once they're identified.

Identifying communication patterns:

43. "What typically happens when you try to discuss difficult topics?"
44. "How do your conversations about problems usually go?"
45. "Who tends to bring up issues? How does the other person typically respond?"
46. "What happens when emotions get high during discussions?"
47. "How do you each handle conflict in your relationship?"
48. "What communication patterns do you recognize from your families of origin?"

Reflecting problematic patterns:

49. "You start conversations hoping to connect, but they often end in arguments."
50. "One of you pursues discussion while the other withdraws, which frustrates you both."
51. "You both care deeply, but you show it in ways that the other person experiences as criticism."
52. "Your attempts to solve problems sometimes create new problems."
53. "You're both trying to protect yourselves, but it's creating distance between you."

Addressing Emotional Safety

Before couples can work on specific issues, they need to feel emotionally safe with each other. This might require addressing patterns of criticism, contempt, defensiveness, or emotional withdrawal.

Exploring emotional safety:

54. "What makes you feel safe to be vulnerable with [partner]?"
55. "When do you feel most guarded or defensive in your relationship?"
56. "What would help you trust that it's safe to share your feelings?"
57. "How do you know when [partner] is really listening to you?"
58. "What shuts you down during difficult conversations?"
59. "What helps you stay open when discussions get heated?"

When safety has been damaged:

60. "Trust has been broken, and rebuilding it will take time."
61. "You're both being careful with each other, which makes sense given what's happened."
62. "You want to be close, but you're also protecting yourselves from more hurt."
63. "It's hard to work on problems when you don't feel emotionally safe."
64. "You both need evidence that things can be different before you'll fully invest in change."

Working with Affairs and Betrayals

Infidelity and other betrayals create specific challenges requiring specialized responses. The betrayed partner needs validation and safety, while the partner who betrayed needs accountability without shame that prevents change.

Responding to betrayal:

65. "This betrayal has shattered your trust and sense of safety."
66. "You're dealing with shock, anger, and grief all at once."
67. "You need to know that [partner] understands the full impact of what happened."

68. "Rebuilding trust will require consistent actions over time, not just words."
69. "You have every right to feel angry and hurt about what happened."

Working with the betraying partner:

70. "You're dealing with guilt and shame about choices you made."
71. "You want to make this right, but you're not sure how."
72. "Your actions have consequences that extend beyond what you intended."
73. "Taking full responsibility without making excuses is the first step."
74. "You'll need to be patient as [partner] works through their feelings."

Exploring Commitment and Motivation

Not all couples are equally committed to working on their relationship. Some people are motivated to change while others are considering leaving. Understanding each person's commitment level helps guide your approach.

Assessing commitment:

75. "How committed do you feel to working on this relationship?"
76. "What would need to change for you to feel hopeful about your future together?"
77. "What makes you want to keep trying versus wanting to give up?"
78. "How do you each feel about the amount of effort required to improve things?"
79. "What would success look like for you in terms of your relationship?"

When commitment differs:

80. "You're both here, but you have different levels of hope about whether things can improve."
81. "One of you is ready to fight for the relationship while the other is considering whether it's worth saving."
82. "You're in different places in terms of how much energy you want to invest in change."
83. "Your different commitment levels are part of what you'll need to work through."

Parenting and Co-Parenting Issues

When couples have children, relationship problems affect the whole family. Parenting disagreements can create additional conflict, and children may be caught in the middle.

Addressing parenting conflicts:

84. "You have different ideas about how to handle parenting situations."
85. "Your children are affected by the tension between you, even when you try to hide it."
86. "You both want what's best for your kids, but you disagree about what that looks like."
87. "Parenting is harder when you're not united as a team."
88. "Your kids need you to work together, even if your relationship is struggling."

Co-parenting after separation:

89. "Your relationship as partners may be ending, but your relationship as co-parents will continue."
90. "You can disagree about your marriage and still agree about what's best for your children."
91. "Your kids need both of you, even if you can't be together."
92. "How you handle this transition will affect your children for years to come."

Working with Extended Family Issues

In-laws, parents, and other extended family members can create stress in relationships. Couples need to learn how to set boundaries while maintaining important family connections.

Addressing family-of-origin issues:

93. "Your families have different ways of handling [situations], and that creates conflict for you."
94. "You feel caught between your partner and your family."
95. "Extended family involvement is affecting your relationship with each other."
96. "You need to figure out how to honor your families while prioritizing your relationship."
97. "Old family patterns are playing out in your marriage."

Financial and Practical Stressors

Money, household responsibilities, and other practical issues can create or worsen relationship problems. These concrete issues often represent deeper dynamics about control, fairness, and priorities.

Addressing practical conflicts:

98. "Money disagreements are about more than just dollars—they're about values and control."
99. "You have different ideas about fairness when it comes to household responsibilities."
100. "Financial stress is affecting your relationship and your individual well-being."
101. "You need to find ways to make practical decisions together without constant conflict."
102. "These day-to-day issues matter because they affect how valued and respected you feel."

Intimacy and Physical Connection

Many couples struggle with mismatched desires for physical and emotional intimacy. These conversations require sensitivity and recognition that intimacy needs vary widely between individuals.

Discussing intimacy:

103.   "You have different needs when it comes to physical closeness."
104.   "Intimacy involves more than just sex—it's about feeling connected and desired."
105.   "You both want to feel wanted, but you express and receive that differently."
106.   "Physical intimacy is affected by emotional connection and relationship satisfaction."
107.   "You need to feel emotionally safe before you can be physically vulnerable."

When intimacy has declined:

108.   "You miss the physical connection you used to have."
109.   "Life stresses and relationship problems have affected your intimate relationship."
110.   "You're both feeling rejected, just in different ways."
111.   "Rebuilding physical intimacy might require working on emotional intimacy first."

Considering Separation and Divorce

Some couples need to explore whether their relationship can be saved or whether separation is the healthiest choice. This requires honest assessment without pushing people toward any particular outcome.

Exploring relationship viability:

112.   "You're both questioning whether this relationship can work long-term."
113.   "You want to know if you've tried everything before making a final decision."
114.   "Some problems can be solved, and others might be fundamental incompatibilities."
115.   "You need to decide if the relationship you can realistically have together is good enough for both of you."
116.   "Sometimes loving someone means recognizing when the relationship isn't healthy for either of you."

When separation seems likely:

117.   "If you do decide to separate, how do you want to handle it in a way that honors what you've meant to each other?"
118.   "You can end your romantic relationship while still treating each other with respect."
119.   "Even if your marriage doesn't work, you can avoid destroying each other in the process."
120.   "How you separate will affect your ability to co-parent and move forward with your lives."

The Challenge of Neutral Alliance

In relationship work, your biggest challenge is maintaining alliance with everyone while not taking sides. Each person needs to feel understood and supported without feeling like you agree with their version of events over their partner's.

This requires constant attention to balance in your reflections, equal time and energy for each person's concerns, and careful language that validates experience without confirming interpretations. When you succeed in this balance, you create space for couples to hear each other in new ways and find solutions that work for everyone.

The goal isn't to save every relationship, but to help each couple make conscious, informed decisions about their future together.

Sometimes the most loving thing people can do is recognize when a relationship has run its course and end it with as much kindness and respect as possible.

Chapter 12: Career and Life Transitions - Major Change Discussions

Life transitions—changing careers, retiring, becoming a parent, dealing with empty nest, moving, ending relationships—create unique counseling challenges. Unlike other issues where the goal is often to solve a problem, transitions involve moving from one life stage or identity to another. This process can be exciting, terrifying, or both simultaneously.

Transitions often involve grief for what's being left behind, anxiety about the unknown future, and confusion about identity. Someone might know they need to make a change but feel paralyzed by the possibilities or overwhelmed by the steps required. Others might be forced into transitions by circumstances beyond their control.

Your role is to help people navigate the emotional complexity of change while supporting them in making decisions that align with their values and goals. This requires understanding both the practical and psychological aspects of major life changes.

Opening Transition Conversations

People facing major life changes often feel pressure to make decisions quickly or move in directions that others expect. Your opening needs to create space for honest exploration without assumptions about what they should do.

Transition-friendly openings:

1. "Tell me about the changes you're considering/facing in your life."
2. "What's bringing this decision to the forefront for you right now?"
3. "How are you feeling about this transition you're going through?"
4. "What's it like to be at this crossroads in your life?"
5. "What thoughts and feelings come up when you think about making this change?"
6. "What made you start thinking about changing [career/relationship/living situation]?"
7. "How long have you been considering this transition?"
8. "What would be helpful to explore about this decision?"

These openings acknowledge that the person is in a process of change without rushing them toward any particular outcome.

Exploring What's Driving the Need for Change

Understanding what's motivating someone to consider a major change helps clarify whether they're moving toward something positive or running away from something negative. Both can be valid motivations, but they require different approaches.

Understanding change motivation:

9. "What's pushing you toward making this change right now?"
10. "What would happen if you didn't make any changes and stayed with the status quo?"
11. "What's not working about your current situation?"
12. "What are you hoping to gain by making this transition?"
13. "What would you lose if you stayed in your current situation long-term?"
14. "How long have you felt like something needed to change?"

Moving toward versus moving away:

15. "Are you more excited about where you're going or relieved about what you're leaving?"
16. "You seem to be running away from problems rather than running toward opportunities."
17. "You have a clear vision of what you don't want, but what do you want?"
18. "You're escaping something painful, and you're also moving toward something hopeful."

Research on approach versus avoidance motivation shows that moving toward positive goals tends to be more sustainable than moving away from negative situations (Elliot, 2008). Understanding this distinction helps guide the conversation.

Working with Career Transitions

Career changes involve practical considerations like finances and logistics, but also identity issues about purpose, achievement, and self-worth. Many people derive significant identity from their work, making career transitions feel like identity crises.

Exploring career dissatisfaction:

19. "What's not working about your current job/career?"
20. "How has your relationship with work changed over time?"
21. "What do you miss about work that you used to enjoy?"
22. "How is your current job affecting other areas of your life?"
23. "What would need to change for you to feel satisfied in your current role?"
24. "When do you feel most engaged and energized at work?"

Exploring career aspirations:

25. "What would your ideal work situation look like?"
26. "What kind of work would make you excited to get up in the morning?"
27. "What skills and talents do you want to use more in your career?"

28. "What impact do you want your work to have on others?"
29. "How important is [money/recognition/flexibility/creativity] to you in work?"
30. "What would make you feel proud of your professional life?"

Identity and Role Changes

Major transitions often involve changes in identity and social roles. Someone retiring may struggle with no longer being a "professional." A new parent might feel lost without their previous identity. These identity shifts can be disorienting.

Exploring identity concerns:

31. "Who are you when you're not a [previous role]?"
32. "How do you introduce yourself when your old identity no longer fits?"
33. "What parts of your identity feel stable even as other parts are changing?"
34. "You're grieving the loss of who you used to be while figuring out who you're becoming."
35. "This transition is changing not just what you do but how you see yourself."

Supporting identity development:

36. "You're more than any single role you play in life."
37. "You get to decide who you want to become in this next chapter."
38. "Your core values and character remain the same even as your circumstances change."
39. "This is an opportunity to rediscover parts of yourself that got buried."
40. "You're not starting from zero—you're building on everything you've already learned and become."

Managing Transition Anxiety

The unknown nature of transitions creates anxiety for most people. They might worry about making the wrong choice, failing in a new situation, or not being able to handle the challenges ahead.

Acknowledging transition fears:

41. "There's something scary about leaving the familiar, even when it's not perfect."
42. "You're worried about making the wrong choice and regretting it later."
43. "The unknown feels risky compared to the problems you know how to handle."
44. "You're afraid you might not be capable of succeeding in this new situation."
45. "It's frightening to give up security for possibility."
46. "What if you make this big change and it doesn't turn out the way you hope?"

Normalizing transition anxiety:

47. "Most people feel anxious about major life changes, even positive ones."
48. "Being nervous about a big transition shows that you're taking it seriously."
49. "You can be excited and scared at the same time."
50. "Anxiety often comes with any decision that really matters to you."
51. "The biggest regrets usually come from chances not taken rather than changes that didn't work out perfectly."

Financial and Practical Concerns

Major life changes often involve financial risks or practical complications. These concrete concerns can't be ignored, but they also shouldn't automatically override other considerations.

Addressing practical concerns:

52. "How would this change affect your financial security?"
53. "What practical steps would need to happen to make this transition possible?"
54. "What's the worst-case scenario if things don't work out as planned?"
55. "How much financial risk feels acceptable to you?"
56. "What would you need to have in place to feel secure about making this change?"
57. "How could you minimize the practical risks while still pursuing the change?"

Balancing security and risk:

58. "You're weighing financial security against personal fulfillment."
59. "You want to be responsible, but you also don't want to live with regret."
60. "Some risks are worth taking, and others aren't."
61. "You're trying to make a smart decision, not just a safe one."
62. "Perfect security doesn't exist, so you're deciding what level of risk is acceptable."

Family and Relationship Impact

Major life transitions affect entire family systems. Spouses, children, and extended family members all have opinions and concerns about big changes. Balancing personal needs with family considerations requires careful thought.

Exploring family impact:

63. "How is your family responding to your desire to make this change?"
64. "What concerns do the important people in your life have about this transition?"

65. "How would this change affect your spouse/children/parents?"
66. "What support do you need from your family to make this work?"
67. "How do you balance what you need for yourself with what's best for your family?"

When family opposes the change:

68. "Your family wants you to be happy, but they're also worried about the risks."
69. "The people who love you might have a hard time supporting changes that feel risky to them."
70. "You need your family's support, but you also need to make choices that are right for your life."
71. "Sometimes you have to disappoint others in the short term to create long-term satisfaction."
72. "Your family's concerns come from love, even if they don't feel supportive."

Timing and Readiness

Knowing when to make a major life change is one of the most difficult aspects of transitions. Some people move too quickly without adequate preparation. Others wait so long for the "perfect" time that they never make the change.

Exploring timing concerns:

73. "What makes this feel like the right time for this change?"
74. "What would you need to see or feel to know you're ready?"
75. "Are you waiting for the perfect moment, or are you avoiding the decision?"
76. "What's the cost of waiting longer versus the cost of moving too quickly?"
77. "What signs would tell you that you've waited too long?"
78. "How will you know when you've prepared enough?"

When timing feels off:

79. "Something doesn't feel quite right about the timing, even though you want to make this change."
80. "You're eager to move forward, but part of you thinks you should wait."
81. "There might never be a perfect time, but some times are better than others."
82. "You can take steps toward change without making the final commitment today."
83. "Preparation and action can happen simultaneously."

Dealing with Regret and "What If" Thinking

Transitions often bring up regrets about past decisions and anxiety about future "what ifs." This mental time travel can prevent people from making decisions based on current realities and future possibilities.

Addressing regret:

84. "You're looking back at choices you made and wondering how things might have been different."
85. "Some regret is normal when you're considering major changes."
86. "You can't change the past, but you can learn from it as you make current decisions."
87. "The person you were then made the best decisions they could with what they knew."
88. "Regret can be information about what you want to do differently going forward."

Managing "what if" anxiety:

89. "You're trying to predict and control outcomes that are ultimately unknowable."
90. "What if it works out better than you can imagine right now?"

91. "You can't eliminate all risk, but you can prepare for likely scenarios."
92. "Some questions can only be answered by taking action."
93. "The biggest risk might be not taking any risk at all."

Supporting Decision-Making

Rather than telling people what to do, your job is to help them access their own wisdom and make decisions that align with their values and goals.

Decision-making support:

94. "What does your gut tell you about this decision?"
95. "If you knew you couldn't fail, what would you choose?"
96. "What would you regret more—trying and failing, or never trying at all?"
97. "What would 80-year-old you want current you to do?"
98. "If your best friend was in this exact situation, what would you advise them?"
99. "What decision would you make if you were only considering yourself?"
100. "What choice would make the best story to tell later?"

When decisions feel overwhelming:

101. "You don't have to figure out the entire path—just the next step."
102. "Some decisions can be reversed or adjusted if they don't work out."
103. "You're making the best decision you can with the information you have now."
104. "Perfect clarity isn't required to make good choices."
105. "Sometimes you have to act your way into a new way of thinking."

Retirement Transitions

Retirement represents a major identity shift from "worker" to something else. Many people struggle with loss of purpose, routine, and social connections that work provided.

Retirement-specific concerns:

106.   "Work has provided structure and purpose for most of your adult life."
107.   "You're excited about freedom from work stress, but also worried about losing meaning."
108.   "Your professional identity has been so central that retirement feels like losing yourself."
109.   "You've been so focused on career that you're not sure what else interests you."
110.   "Retirement isn't just about stopping work—it's about starting something new."
111.   "You have decades of experience and wisdom to contribute in new ways."

When retirement is forced:

112.   "You weren't ready to retire, but circumstances made the decision for you."
113.   "This feels like loss rather than opportunity right now."
114.   "You're grieving the end of your career while trying to figure out what comes next."
115.   "Forced retirement can become chosen opportunity with time."

Relationship Transitions

Ending marriages, starting new relationships, or dealing with children leaving home all involve changes in primary relationships that affect daily life and identity.

Divorce and separation:

116.   "Ending this relationship means rebuilding your entire life structure."
117.   "You're grieving not just the relationship, but the future you thought you'd have."
118.   "You're scared about being alone, but also excited about the possibility of being yourself."
119.   "This decision affects every aspect of your life— where you live, your finances, your daily routine."
120.   "You can mourn the end of your marriage while still knowing it was the right choice."

New relationships:

121.   "Starting over in love feels both hopeful and terrifying."
122.   "You want to be open to love, but you're also protecting yourself from getting hurt again."
123.   "This relationship represents possibility, but also risk."
124.   "You're trying to learn from past relationships while not letting them limit your future."

Empty Nest and Parenting Transitions

When children leave home or become independent, parents face identity shifts from active parenting to whatever comes next.

Empty nest transitions:

125.   "Your primary job for [years] has been raising children, and that phase is ending."
126.   "You're proud of raising independent kids, but also sad about them not needing you the same way."
127.   "You and your spouse need to rediscover who you are as a couple, not just as parents."

128. "This is an opportunity to reconnect with interests and dreams you put on hold."
129. "You're not losing your children—you're gaining adult relationships with them."

Geographic and Living Situation Changes

Moving to new locations or changing living situations involves practical adjustments and often social and emotional challenges.

Relocation concerns:

130. "Moving means leaving behind familiar places and established relationships."
131. "You're excited about new opportunities, but also anxious about starting over socially."
132. "This move is necessary for [career/family/finances], but it still feels like loss."
133. "You're worried about whether you'll be able to create the same sense of community in a new place."

Creating Action Plans

Once someone has clarity about what they want to change, they need concrete steps to move forward. Your role is to help them break down overwhelming transitions into manageable actions.

Planning for action:

134. "What would be the very first step you'd need to take?"
135. "How could you test out this change in a small way before making the full commitment?"
136. "What information do you need to gather before you can move forward?"
137. "Who could you talk to who has made a similar transition?"

138.	"What would need to happen in the next month for you to feel like you're making progress?"
139.	"How will you know if this change is working out the way you hope?"

When action feels overwhelming:

140.	"You don't have to do everything at once—just something."
141.	"Movement in any direction is better than staying stuck."
142.	"You can take one step and then reassess before taking the next one."
143.	"Progress doesn't have to be fast to be meaningful."
144.	"Every small action builds momentum toward the bigger change."

Maintaining Perspective During Transitions

Major life changes can feel all-consuming. Helping clients maintain perspective prevents them from making decisions based on temporary emotions or losing sight of their broader life context.

Perspective-maintaining responses:

145.	"This transition is important, but it's not your entire life story."
146.	"You've successfully navigated major changes before."
147.	"The anxiety you're feeling now is temporary, even though the change might be permanent."
148.	"This decision matters, but it's not irreversible if it doesn't work out."
149.	"You have more resources and wisdom now than you had during previous transitions."
150.	"This change is one chapter in your life, not the whole book."

The Gift of Transitions

While transitions can be stressful and uncertain, they also represent opportunities for growth, renewal, and alignment with evolving values and priorities. Your role is to help clients navigate the challenges while remaining open to the possibilities that change can bring.

The most successful transitions happen when people connect with their own motivations for change, prepare thoughtfully for the practical realities, and maintain support systems during the process. When you help someone approach a major life change with both excitement and realistic planning, you're supporting them in creating a life that reflects who they're becoming, not just who they've been.

Adapting to Every Situation

These situation-specific scripts demonstrate how the core principles of MI translate across different contexts and populations. While the underlying approach remains consistent—curiosity, respect, collaboration—the specific language and concerns adapt to meet people exactly where they are.

The next section explores the advanced MI techniques that experienced practitioners use to navigate complex situations, handle resistance, and help clients move from contemplation to committed action. These are the skills that separate competent MI practitioners from true artists of change conversation.

Part IV: Advanced Techniques

The techniques in this final section represent the advanced artistry of Motivational Interviewing. While anyone can learn to reflect and affirm, these skills require nuanced judgment, perfect timing, and deep understanding of human psychology. They're the difference between competent MI practice and transformational conversations that create lasting change.

These advanced techniques—developing discrepancy, rolling with resistance, and evoking commitment—require you to dance on the edge of challenge and support. Too little challenge and clients stay comfortable in their problems. Too much and they become defensive or shut down. The art is finding that sweet spot where people feel supported enough to be honest about difficult truths.

Mastering these skills takes time and practice. They require not just knowing what to say, but when to say it, how to say it, and when to say nothing at all. They're about reading between the lines, sensing what's unspoken, and creating the conditions where people talk themselves into change.

Chapter 13: Developing Discrepancy - Gentle Confrontation Phrases

Developing discrepancy is perhaps the most sophisticated skill in Motivational Interviewing. It involves helping clients recognize the gaps between their current behaviors and their stated values, goals, or desired outcomes. The challenge is doing this in a way that creates motivation rather than defensiveness.

Most people live with some level of cognitive dissonance—they know what they should do but continue doing something different. They value health but smoke cigarettes. They want close relationships but behave in ways that push people away. They claim family is their priority but work constantly. This internal conflict creates psychological tension that can either be ignored through rationalization or used as fuel for change.

Your job isn't to point out these discrepancies like a prosecutor presenting evidence. Instead, you help clients discover these gaps for themselves through careful questioning and reflection. When people recognize their own inconsistencies, they're much more likely to do something about them than when someone else points them out.

The Art of Gentle Confrontation

Confrontation in MI doesn't mean being aggressive or accusatory. It means placing conflicting pieces of information side by side and letting the client make sense of the discrepancy. Think of it as holding up two mirrors so someone can see themselves from different angles.

Basic discrepancy reflections:

1. "On one hand you say family is your highest priority, and on the other hand you're working 70 hours a week."

2. "You want to be healthy, and you're also continuing behaviors that put your health at risk."
3. "You value honesty, but you're finding yourself lying to cover up your drinking."
4. "You say you want to lose weight, but you keep making food choices that take you in the opposite direction."
5. "Being a good parent matters to you, and your kids are telling you they're worried about your behavior."
6. "You want people to trust you, but you keep breaking promises to yourself and others."

These reflections present the discrepancy without judgment, allowing clients to wrestle with the contradiction rather than defend against an attack.

Highlighting Value-Behavior Discrepancies

The most powerful discrepancies involve core values because people generally can't tolerate acting against their fundamental beliefs for extended periods.

Values-based discrepancy responses:

7. "Help me understand how using drugs fits with your image of yourself as a responsible person."
8. "You've described yourself as someone who always follows through on commitments, but you're struggling to keep commitments to yourself about your health."
9. "Being authentic is really important to you, but right now you're living a life that doesn't feel genuine."
10. "You pride yourself on being in control, but this behavior is controlling you."
11. "Independence matters to you, but you're becoming dependent on something you don't want to need."
12. "You want to be someone your children can be proud of. How does your current situation fit with that goal?"

Research shows that value-behavior discrepancies create more motivation for change than other types of inconsistencies because they threaten core identity (Rokeach, 1973). When behavior conflicts with deeply held values, psychological pressure for change increases.

Present-Future Discrepancy Development

This technique involves helping clients see how their current path conflicts with their desired future.

Future-focused discrepancy statements:

13. "You have goals for where you want to be in five years, but your current choices are taking you in a different direction."
14. "The person you want to become and the person you're being right now seem like different people."
15. "You're dreaming of a future that your current behavior makes less likely."
16. "If you continue on this path, where do you see yourself ending up?"
17. "Your vision for your life and your current reality don't match up."
18. "You're hoping for changes in your life while continuing patterns that prevent those changes."

When exploring consequences:

19. "What you're doing now might feel manageable, but where does this road lead?"
20. "You're handling the current problems your behavior creates, but what happens if things get worse?"
21. "Right now you can still choose. At what point might that choice be taken away?"
22. "You're maintaining control now, but how long can you keep all these balls in the air?"

Past-Present Discrepancies

Sometimes clients need to recognize how much they've changed from who they used to be or wanted to be.

Comparing past and present:

23. "The person you used to be wouldn't recognize the person you are today."
24. "You've told me about who you were before this problem started. What happened to that person?"
25. "You had dreams and plans that seem to have gotten lost along the way."
26. "There was a time when you would never have imagined yourself in this situation."
27. "You used to have standards for yourself that you're not meeting anymore."
28. "The younger version of you had hopes that the current version isn't pursuing."

When clients have lost ground:

29. "You've worked hard to build something, and now you're watching it slip away."
30. "The progress you made before shows you're capable of more than what you're doing now."
31. "You know what it feels like to be proud of yourself, and that feeling seems distant now."
32. "You've proven you can change before. What's different this time?"

Exploring the Costs of Status Quo

Sometimes discrepancy involves helping clients recognize what they're giving up by not changing.

Cost-focused discrepancy development:

33. "What are you losing by continuing this pattern?"
34. "While you're maintaining this behavior, what opportunities are passing you by?"
35. "The price of staying the same is getting higher."
36. "What would you gain if this problem disappeared tomorrow?"
37. "You're paying a cost for every day you don't address this issue."
38. "This situation is stealing things from you that you can't get back."

When change feels risky:

39. "You're weighing the risks of changing against the risks of not changing."
40. "What feels safe in the short term might be dangerous in the long term."
41. "You're protecting yourself from the uncertainty of change, but what's the cost of certainty?"
42. "The devil you know might be more dangerous than the devil you don't know."

Working with Rationalization and Denial

When clients minimize problems or make excuses, discrepancy development can gently challenge their defenses without attacking them directly.

Addressing minimization:

43. "You say it's not that bad, but it brought you to counseling."
44. "If this isn't a big deal, what made you think you needed help?"
45. "You describe this as minor, but it seems to be affecting major areas of your life."
46. "For something that's not a problem, it sure takes up a lot of your mental energy."

47. "You're handling it fine, except for [list the areas where it's not fine]."

When clients make excuses:

48. "You have reasons for your behavior, and you also have reasons for wanting to change."
49. "Your explanations make sense, but they don't change the consequences you're experiencing."
50. "Understanding why you do something doesn't eliminate the need to consider whether you want to keep doing it."
51. "You can be right about your reasons and still be wrong about whether this is working for you."

Highlighting Contradictory Statements

Sometimes clients present conflicting information within the same conversation. Gently highlighting these contradictions can increase awareness.

Pointing out contradictions:

52. "A few minutes ago you said [one thing], but now you're saying [contradictory thing]. Help me understand."
53. "Earlier you mentioned that [behavior] wasn't a problem, but you also described [consequences]. How do those fit together?"
54. "You've said both that you're in control and that you feel out of control. What's that about?"
55. "Part of what you're telling me suggests things are fine, but part suggests you're concerned."
56. "You seem to have mixed feelings about whether this is actually a problem."

Using Hypothetical Scenarios

Hypothetical questions can help clients explore discrepancies without feeling directly confronted.

Hypothetical discrepancy exploration:

57. "If your best friend was doing exactly what you're doing, what would you tell them?"
58. "What would someone who cares about you say about this situation?"
59. "If you knew for certain that continuing this behavior would cost you [important thing], what would you do?"
60. "Imagine explaining your current choices to your children when they're adults. How would that conversation go?"
61. "If you could see yourself from the outside, what would you notice?"

Future self scenarios:

62. "What would 80-year-old you want current you to know?"
63. "If you could send a message back from the future, what would you tell yourself?"
64. "When you're old and looking back on this time in your life, what would you want to see?"
65. "How will you feel about these choices a year from now?"

Amplifying Natural Consequences

Rather than threatening consequences, you can help clients recognize consequences they're already experiencing or logically heading toward.

Natural consequence awareness:

66. "You mentioned that [consequence] happened. How does that connect to [behavior]?"
67. "What do you make of the fact that every time you [behavior], [consequence] follows?"
68. "You're seeing a pattern where [behavior] leads to [result]. What's your take on that?"
69. "The consequences you're describing seem to be escalating over time."

70. "What started as a small problem seems to be growing into a bigger one."

When consequences seem distant:

71. "The effects might not be visible today, but they're building up."
72. "Some consequences show up immediately, others take time to develop."
73. "You're taking out a loan against your future, and the interest is compounding."
74. "What looks manageable now might become unmanageable later."

Exploring the Effort Required to Maintain Status Quo

Sometimes people don't realize how much energy they're putting into maintaining problematic patterns.

Effort-based discrepancy development:

75. "How much time and energy does it take to manage this problem?"
76. "You're working really hard to keep this from getting worse, but wouldn't it be easier to make it better?"
77. "All the effort you put into hiding/managing/controlling this could be used for something else."
78. "You're exhausted from trying to keep everything together."
79. "What would you do with all that mental space if you weren't constantly thinking about this issue?"

When clients are tired:

80. "You sound worn out from trying to balance everything."
81. "The energy you spend on this problem could be energy you spend on your goals."

82. "You're managing a crisis that could become a solution with different choices."
83. "All this effort to stay the same—imagine what you could accomplish if you put that energy toward change."

Working with Perfectionism and High Standards

High-achieving clients often struggle with discrepancies between their standards and their current behavior.

Standards-based discrepancy work:

84. "You have high standards for yourself in other areas. How does this situation fit with those standards?"
85. "You're someone who usually excels, but you're accepting mediocrity in this area."
86. "Excellence matters to you everywhere except here. What's different about this?"
87. "You wouldn't tolerate this level of performance from others, but you're tolerating it from yourself."
88. "Your reputation for reliability is important to you, but you're being unreliable to yourself."

Using Client's Own Expertise

Many clients are experts in areas where the same principles apply to their current problem.

Expertise-based discrepancy development:

89. "In your profession, you wouldn't accept this level of [inefficiency/risk/inconsistency]. What makes this situation different?"
90. "You give great advice to others about [related area]. What would you tell yourself?"

91. "You're successful in [area] because you [positive qualities]. How could those same qualities help here?"
92. "You know what it takes to solve problems because you do it all the time. What's stopping you from applying that here?"
93. "You're an expert at [skill]. How does that expertise translate to this situation?"

The Timing of Discrepancy Development

Developing discrepancy requires exquisite timing. Too early in the relationship and clients feel attacked. Too late and they may have already convinced themselves that change isn't necessary. The sweet spot is usually after rapport has been established but before clients have built up too many defenses.

Watch for signs that clients are ready for gentle confrontation: they've expressed some concern about their situation, they've acknowledged that change might be helpful, or they've shared information that reveals contradictions. These moments create openings for discrepancy development.

Also watch for signs that clients aren't ready: they're highly defensive, they haven't acknowledged any problems, or they seem fragile or overwhelmed. Pushing discrepancy too hard or too early can damage the therapeutic relationship.

Avoiding the Traps

The biggest trap in discrepancy development is becoming invested in making the client see their contradictions. When you're working harder than they are to recognize the discrepancy, you've crossed from MI into confrontation. The goal is to plant seeds of awareness, not to force immediate recognition.

Another trap is using discrepancy development to prove a point or win an argument. The purpose isn't to be right about the client's situation but to help them gain clarity about their own motivations and barriers.

Some clients will recognize discrepancies but not be ready to change. That's normal and acceptable. Awareness often precedes action by weeks, months, or even years. Your job is to support the awareness process without demanding immediate behavior change.

The Dance Between Challenge and Support

The most effective discrepancy development happens in the context of a supportive relationship. Clients need to feel that you're on their side, trying to help them understand themselves better rather than criticizing their choices.

This means balancing every discrepancy development with affirmation and empathy. "You have high standards for yourself, and you're struggling with not meeting them in this area" combines challenge with understanding. "You care so much about your family that it's painful to see how your behavior is affecting them" acknowledges both the discrepancy and the positive values driving their concern.

The goal is to help clients become curious about their own contradictions rather than defensive about them. When someone feels supported and understood, they're much more likely to look honestly at uncomfortable truths about themselves.

Moving from Awareness to Action

Developing discrepancy creates psychological tension that can fuel motivation for change. But awareness alone doesn't create change— it creates readiness for change. Once clients recognize important discrepancies, your job shifts to helping them explore what they might want to do about them.

Some clients will immediately want to make changes once they see important contradictions. Others will need time to sit with the awareness before they're ready for action. Both responses are normal and workable.

The most important thing is that the recognition of discrepancy comes from the client, not from you. When people discover their own contradictions, they own the awareness and are more likely to act on it. When contradictions are pointed out by others, people often feel defensive and work harder to justify their behavior rather than change it.

Chapter 14: Rolling with Resistance - Aikido-Inspired Responses

Resistance in counseling is like water flowing downhill—it follows the path of least resistance and finds ways around obstacles. When you push against it directly, it pushes back. When you try to stop it, it builds pressure until it breaks through. But when you learn to work with its natural flow, resistance becomes a source of energy that can be redirected toward positive change.

The martial art of Aikido offers a perfect metaphor for handling resistance. Rather than meeting force with force, Aikido practitioners use an opponent's energy and momentum to redirect the attack. They blend with incoming force and guide it in a new direction. This same principle transforms resistance from an obstacle into an opportunity.

In MI, rolling with resistance means accepting and working with client ambivalence rather than fighting against it. It means joining with the resistant part of the client while gently guiding the conversation toward change. Most importantly, it means understanding that resistance often contains valuable information about what clients need to feel safe enough to change.

Understanding What Resistance Really Means

Resistance isn't defiance or stubbornness (though it might look that way). It's usually a signal that something about the change process feels unsafe, overwhelming, or inconsistent with the client's values or identity. Resistance is often protection, not obstruction.

When someone argues against change, they might be protecting their autonomy, their self-image, or their coping mechanisms. When they minimize problems, they might be protecting themselves from feeling overwhelmed by the scope of necessary changes. When they make excuses, they might be protecting their self-worth from the shame of admitting failure.

Understanding resistance as protection changes how you respond to it. Instead of seeing it as something to overcome, you see it as information about what the client needs to feel safe enough to change.

The Classic Aikido Response

The most basic Aikido response involves agreement with the resistant statement followed by a gentle redirection. You blend with the client's energy and then guide it in a slightly different direction.

Basic Aikido responses:

1. "You're absolutely right that no one can force you to change. What changes, if any, would you choose for yourself?"
2. "You know yourself better than anyone else. What do you think would work for you?"
3. "That's true—this is completely your decision. What's appealing to you about staying the same versus changing?"
4. "You're right that change is hard. What would make it worth the difficulty for you?"
5. "Exactly—you've managed this long without help. What's different now that made you consider getting support?"
6. "You're correct that I don't understand your situation the way you do. Help me understand what's most important."

These responses validate the client's autonomy while opening space for exploration of their own motivations.

Rolling with "I Don't Have a Problem"

When clients deny or minimize problems, the natural response is to argue or provide evidence of the problem. This almost always increases resistance. Instead, you can agree with their perspective while exploring what brought them to counseling.

Responses to problem denial:

7. "You might be right that this isn't as big a problem as other people think. What made you decide to come talk to someone?"
8. "Maybe it's not a problem for you. What do you think other people are seeing that concerns them?"
9. "It sounds like you're handling things fine from your perspective. What would need to change for you to see it differently?"
10. "You know your situation best. What would have to happen for you to think you needed help?"
11. "That's possible—maybe this isn't the right time to worry about this. What would make it the right time?"
12. "You're managing everything okay right now. What concerns you about the future if things continue as they are?"

When others are concerned:

13. "So other people think there's a problem, but you don't. What do you make of that difference in perspective?"
14. "It sounds like you're getting pressure from people who care about you. How does that feel?"
15. "Your family/employer/court sees this differently than you do. What's that like for you?"
16. "People who matter to you are worried, even though you don't think they need to be. What would help them understand your perspective?"

Working with "I Can't Change"

When clients express helplessness or inability to change, arguing that they can change usually backfires. Instead, you can explore what makes change feel impossible while looking for exceptions and resources.

Responses to "can't" statements:

17. "Change feels impossible right now. What would need to be different for it to feel possible?"
18. "You've tried before and it didn't work. What did you learn from those attempts?"
19. "It seems overwhelming when you look at everything that would need to change. What would be the smallest possible first step?"
20. "You feel stuck in patterns that are bigger than you. What helped you make other difficult changes in your life?"
21. "Right now you can't imagine being different. Tell me about a time when you successfully changed something that seemed impossible."
22. "You're convinced you can't do this. What would prove you wrong?"

When clients feel hopeless:

23. "Hope feels dangerous when you've been disappointed before."
24. "You've tried so many times that it's hard to believe this time would be different."
25. "It makes sense that you'd protect yourself from more disappointment by not trying."
26. "You're tired of setting yourself up for failure."
27. "What if change happened slowly, so slowly you barely noticed it? Would that feel more possible?"

Research on learned helplessness shows that when people believe they have no control, they stop trying even when options become available (Seligman, 1972). Rolling with helplessness while gently exploring past successes can begin to restore a sense of agency.

Handling "I Don't Want to Change"

Sometimes resistance comes from genuine satisfaction with current behavior or fear of what change would cost. These feelings deserve respect and exploration.

Responses to unwillingness:

28. "You like things the way they are. What works about your current situation?"
29. "Change would require giving up things that are important to you."
30. "You've built a life that makes sense to you. What would you be afraid of losing if you changed?"
31. "Maybe the costs of changing feel higher than the costs of staying the same."
32. "You get something valuable from your current patterns. What would you miss most?"
33. "It's smart to be cautious about changes that might make things worse."

When change feels threatening:

34. "Changing might mean becoming someone you're not sure you want to be."
35. "You're comfortable with who you are, even if others aren't comfortable with it."
36. "The devil you know feels safer than the devil you don't know."
37. "You're protecting something important by staying the same."

Rolling with Anger and Hostility

When clients are angry—at you, at the situation, at being required to be there—meeting anger with calmness and curiosity often defuses the intensity.

Responses to anger:

38. "You're really angry about having to be here."
39. "This feels like one more person trying to tell you what to do."
40. "You've had enough of people trying to fix you."
41. "You're mad about losing control over your choices."
42. "It's infuriating when people assume they know what's best for you."
43. "You have every right to be upset about this situation."

When anger masks other emotions:

44. "Underneath all that anger, I'm hearing hurt."
45. "You're angry, and you also sound scared about what might happen."
46. "That anger might be protecting you from feeling vulnerable."
47. "You're pissed off, and you also care deeply about what happens."

Working with Intellectualization and Over-Analysis

Some clients resist change by analyzing everything to death or getting lost in abstract discussions that avoid emotional reality.

Responses to intellectualization:

48. "You understand this issue really well intellectually. What does it feel like emotionally?"

49. "You can analyze this perfectly, but analysis doesn't always lead to change."
50. "Your head gets it, but what's your heart saying?"
51. "Understanding why you do something doesn't automatically change your desire to do it."
52. "You're great at figuring out the 'why' behind your behavior. What about the 'what now'?"

When clients avoid feelings:

53. "You think about this a lot, but talking about thoughts is different from talking about feelings."
54. "Your mind is working hard to solve this, but solutions aren't always logical."
55. "You're very smart about this problem. What does your gut tell you?"
56. "Sometimes the answer isn't in more analysis but in experiencing things differently."

Rolling with Blame and Externalization

When clients blame others for their problems or focus on things outside their control, joining with their frustration while gently redirecting can be more effective than confrontation.

Responses to blame:

57. "Other people's behavior is definitely affecting you. What can you control in this situation?"
58. "You're right that [other person] is being difficult. How do you want to respond to that?"
59. "That person really is causing problems for you. What would you like to be different about how you handle it?"
60. "You can't change them, but you might be able to change how their behavior affects you."
61. "It's frustrating when other people don't do what they should. What are your options for dealing with that?"

When clients feel victimized:

62. "You didn't choose this situation, but you're stuck dealing with it."
63. "Life has handed you some unfair circumstances. How do you want to respond?"
64. "You've been hurt by people and situations beyond your control. What power do you have now?"
65. "This shouldn't be your problem to solve, but it is. What would help?"

Using Amplified Reflection

Sometimes rolling with resistance involves amplifying or overstating the client's position. This can help them hear how extreme their stance sounds and naturally move toward a more moderate position.

Amplified reflections:

66. "So you're saying you never want to change anything about your current situation."
67. "It sounds like you're completely satisfied with how things are going."
68. "You believe there's absolutely nothing problematic about your current patterns."
69. "Change is completely out of the question under any circumstances."
70. "You're convinced that no one could possibly understand your situation."
71. "There's nothing anyone could say that would make you reconsider."

When used carefully, amplified reflections often prompt clients to moderate their statements:

"Well, I didn't say never..." or "I wouldn't go that far..." These responses open space for more nuanced exploration.

Double-Sided Reflections for Resistance

Two-sided reflections acknowledge both the resistant feelings and any change talk that might be present, helping clients see the complexity of their own attitudes.

Double-sided resistance responses:

72. "Part of you is completely done with people telling you what to do, and part of you wonders if they might have a point."
73. "You don't want to change, and you also don't want to keep dealing with the consequences of not changing."
74. "You're comfortable with how you are, and you're also tired of the problems it creates."
75. "You like your life the way it is, and you also see how it's affecting people you care about."
76. "You don't think you need help, and you also recognize that something brought you here."

Coming Alongside Rather Than Opposing

The key to rolling with resistance is positioning yourself as an ally rather than an adversary. You're not trying to convince clients to change—you're helping them explore their own relationship with change.

Collaborative responses:

77. "We're on the same team here. You want what's best for your life."
78. "I'm not here to talk you into anything. I'm here to help you figure out what you want."
79. "You're the expert on your life. I'm just here to ask good questions."
80. "My job isn't to convince you to change. It's to help you think through your options."
81. "You don't have to defend your choices to me. What matters is whether they're working for you."

Working with All-or-Nothing Thinking

When clients think in extremes about change ("I have to be perfect or I'm a failure"), rolling with resistance might involve accepting their perfectionism while exploring alternatives.

Responses to perfectionism:

82. "You hold yourself to really high standards. What would 'good enough' look like?"
83. "You want to do this right or not at all. What would 'right' look like for you?"
84. "Perfection feels necessary, but what if progress was enough?"
85. "You're worried about failing if you can't do this perfectly. What would partial success look like?"
86. "All-or-nothing makes sense when you're tired of half-measures. What would whole-hearted but imperfect effort look like?"

The Paradox of Acceptance

One of the most powerful aspects of rolling with resistance is that when clients feel truly accepted where they are, they often become more open to considering change. When you stop pushing, they stop pushing back.

This doesn't mean you approve of destructive behavior or that you give up hope for positive change. It means you accept that clients have good reasons for their resistance and that change happens on their timeline, not yours.

Acceptance responses:

87. "Maybe now isn't the right time for you to think about changing. What would make it the right time?"
88. "You might decide that the way you're living now is what works for you, and that's your choice to make."

89. "You don't owe anyone change, including me. What would you owe yourself?"
90. "It's possible that staying the same is the right decision for you right now."
91. "You get to choose what changes to make, if any, and when to make them."

Building on Resistance

Sometimes resistance contains seeds of change talk that can be cultivated. When clients argue against change, they often reveal what would need to be different for change to feel acceptable.

Finding change talk in resistance:

92. "You don't want to change because it would mean admitting you have a problem. What would make it okay to have a problem that needs attention?"
93. "You're not ready to change because the timing feels wrong. What would make the timing feel right?"
94. "You don't want help because you value independence. How could getting support actually increase your independence?"
95. "You're resistant to change because past attempts failed. What would need to be different this time?"

The Gentle Redirect

After joining with resistance, the gentle redirect guides the conversation back toward exploration of change without being pushy or manipulative.

Redirection techniques:

96. "You make good points about why change is difficult. What would make it worth the difficulty?"
97. "I hear all the reasons not to change. What reasons, if any, do you have for considering it?"

98. "You're comfortable with things as they are. What would need to shift for you to become uncomfortable with the status quo?"
99. "You don't see problems with your current approach. What would you see as benefits if things were different?"
100. "You have every right to stay exactly as you are. What draws you toward the idea of being different?"

When Rolling Isn't Working

Sometimes rolling with resistance isn't enough. If a client remains highly resistant despite your best efforts, it might be time to step back and examine what's happening in the relationship or what needs aren't being met.

Some resistance is really about the relationship with you rather than about change itself. The client might not feel heard, understood, or respected. Some resistance is about timing—the client might not be ready for change regardless of how skillful your approach.

In these cases, the most helpful thing might be to directly address the resistance: "I notice we keep coming back to all the reasons not to change. What's that about?" or "It seems like part of you doesn't want to be here. Help me understand what would be more helpful."

The Art of Therapeutic Aikido

Rolling with resistance is an art that develops with practice. It requires you to stay calm in the face of hostility, curious in the face of defensiveness, and hopeful in the face of despair. Most importantly, it requires genuine respect for the client's autonomy and wisdom about their own life.

When you master this skill, you transform from someone who argues with clients into someone who helps them argue with themselves. You become a collaborator in their internal dialogue rather than an external force they need to resist. This shift often makes the difference between superficial compliance and genuine commitment to change.

Chapter 15: Commitment - Securing Change Language

Commitment language represents the bridge between thinking about change and actually making change happen. It's the moment when "I should probably" becomes "I will" and "maybe someday" becomes "starting tomorrow." This transition from contemplation to commitment is often the turning point that determines whether someone follows through on their intentions or remains stuck in the cycle of wanting to change without actually changing.

Evoking commitment is different from extracting promises. Promises often feel imposed and create pressure that can backfire. True commitment emerges from internal motivation and feels like a natural next step rather than an obligation to someone else. Your job is to create the conditions where commitment language arises organically from the client's own exploration of their motivations and goals.

The challenge is knowing when and how to invite commitment without pushing for it prematurely. Too early, and you might interrupt the natural process of motivation building. Too late, and the window of opportunity might pass. The art is in recognizing when someone is ready to move from "I want to change" to "I'm going to change" and supporting that transition skillfully.

Recognizing Readiness for Commitment

Before attempting to evoke commitment, you need to recognize signs that someone is psychologically ready to make specific commitments. These signs usually include strong change talk, decreased resistance, clear problem recognition, and specific interest in solutions.

Signs of readiness:

- Client asks what they should do next
- They stop arguing for the status quo
- They express urgency about change
- They start making specific plans spontaneously
- They talk about when rather than if they'll change
- They express confidence in their ability to change
- They stop asking whether they should change and start asking how

When these signs aren't present, your job is to continue building motivation rather than pushing for commitment.

Asking for Commitment Directly

Sometimes the most straightforward approach is simply asking what the client is willing to commit to doing.

Direct commitment requests:

1. "What are you willing to do between now and next time we meet?"
2. "What feels like a realistic commitment you could make to yourself today?"
3. "Given everything we've talked about, what's your next step?"
4. "What would you like to commit to trying this week?"
5. "What specific change are you ready to make?"
6. "What feels like something you could definitely do?"
7. "What commitment would feel challenging but achievable?"
8. "If you were going to take one action based on our conversation, what would it be?"

These direct requests work best when rapport is strong and the client has already expressed motivation for change.

Scaling Questions for Commitment

Scaling questions help clients identify commitments that feel manageable and realistic rather than overwhelming.

Using scales to explore commitment:

9. "On a scale of 1-10, how ready are you to make this change? What would make it a 10?"
10. "If 10 means you're completely committed and 1 means you're not ready at all, where are you right now?"
11. "What would you be willing to commit to on a scale where 10 is everything and 1 is nothing?"
12. "If you had to pick a number between 1-10 for how confident you are that you'll follow through, what would it be?"
13. "On a readiness scale, you said you're a 7. What would you be willing to try that matches that level of readiness?"

Building on scale responses:

14. "You said you're a 6 on readiness. What would a 6-level commitment look like?"
15. "If you're not quite ready for the full change, what partial step matches where you are right now?"
16. "You're somewhere in the middle on commitment. What feels right for someone in the middle?"

Research shows that scaling questions help clients make more realistic commitments because they can choose a level of change that matches their actual readiness (Miller & Rollnick, 2013).

Time-Bound Commitment Exploration

Helping clients think about specific timeframes often makes commitment feel more concrete and achievable.

Time-focused commitment questions:

17. "What could you commit to for the next 24 hours?"
18. "What feels doable between now and next week?"
19. "If you were only committing to today, what would you be willing to try?"
20. "What's a reasonable commitment for the next month?"
21. "What could you do differently tomorrow than you did today?"
22. "If you had to pick just one week to experiment with change, what would you try?"

When long-term change feels overwhelming:

23. "Instead of committing to permanent change, what about committing to a trial period?"
24. "What if you just committed to trying something new for one week?"
25. "Could you commit to change for today and decide about tomorrow when tomorrow comes?"
26. "What feels manageable if you're only thinking about the immediate future?"

Values-Based Commitment Language

The strongest commitments connect to deep personal values rather than external expectations.

Connecting commitment to values:

27. "What commitment would align with who you want to be as a person?"
28. "Given what matters most to you, what feels like the right thing to commit to?"
29. "How can you make a commitment that honors your values?"
30. "What would someone with your values do in this situation?"
31. "What commitment would make you proud of yourself?"

32. "What change would be most consistent with what you believe about yourself?"

When exploring identity and commitment:

33. "The person you want to become would make what kind of commitment?"
34. "What commitment fits with your image of yourself as [positive quality they've mentioned]?"
35. "How can your commitment reflect the best version of yourself?"
36. "What would you commit to if you were already the person you're trying to become?"

Exploring Barriers to Commitment

Sometimes clients hesitate to make commitments because they're aware of obstacles they haven't discussed. Exploring these barriers can lead to more realistic and achievable commitments.

Barrier exploration:

37. "What makes it hard for you to commit to that change?"
38. "What obstacles do you see to following through?"
39. "What would get in the way of you keeping this commitment?"
40. "What concerns you about making this promise to yourself?"
41. "If you made this commitment and then broke it, what would probably have happened?"
42. "What would need to be different for this commitment to feel completely doable?"

Problem-solving around barriers:

43. "How could you work around that obstacle?"
44. "What would help you handle that challenge if it comes up?"
45. "How have you dealt with similar barriers in the past?"
46. "What support would you need to overcome that difficulty?"

47. "If that barrier showed up, what would be your backup plan?"

Strengthening Weak Commitments

Sometimes clients make tentative commitments that sound uncertain. These can often be strengthened through exploration rather than pressure.

Responses to weak commitment language:

48. "You said you'll 'try' to do this. What would help you move from trying to doing?"
49. "I hear some hesitation in your voice about this commitment. What's that about?"
50. "You sound like you're not completely sure about this plan. What would make you more confident?"
51. "What would need to change for this to feel like a definite 'yes' instead of a 'maybe'?"
52. "You're willing to attempt this. What would make the difference between attempting and succeeding?"
53. "I notice you said 'probably.' What would make it 'definitely'?"

When clients hedge their commitments:

54. "You added 'if I can' to your commitment. What might prevent you from being able to?"
55. "You said 'I guess I could try.' What would help you feel more certain?"
56. "There seems to be a 'but' after your commitment. What's the but?"
57. "What would have to happen for you to feel completely committed rather than partially committed?"

Using Change Talk to Build Commitment

When clients express desire, ability, reasons, or need for change, you can use this change talk as a foundation for commitment.

Building on desire statements:

58. "You really want to change this. What are you willing to do about that desire?"
59. "Since you want this so much, what commitment makes sense?"
60. "That wanting sounds strong. How do you want to act on it?"
61. "You've expressed a lot of desire for change. What specific step are you ready to take?"

Building on ability statements:

62. "You think you can do this. What are you willing to commit to trying?"
63. "You have confidence in your ability. How do you want to use that confidence?"
64. "Since you believe you can change this, what will you change?"
65. "You've convinced yourself you're capable. What capability will you put into action?"

Building on reasons:

66. "You have compelling reasons for change. Which reason is strong enough to fuel a commitment?"
67. "Given all the benefits you see in changing, what are you ready to commit to?"
68. "Those are powerful reasons. What action do they point you toward?"

Building on need statements:

69. "You said something has to change. What will you change?"

70. "Since you need to do something different, what specifically will you do?"
71. "You recognize the necessity of change. What necessary step will you take?"

The Importance Ruler for Commitment

This technique helps clients identify what level of commitment matches their level of motivation.

Importance-based commitment questions:

72. "You said this change is important to you. What commitment would match that level of importance?"
73. "If this matters as much as you say it does, what are you willing to do about it?"
74. "How important is this change to you on a scale of 1-10? What's a commitment that fits that level of importance?"
75. "You rated the importance of change as [number]. What's a [number]-level commitment?"
76. "What would someone who cares about this as much as you do commit to doing?"

Confidence-Based Commitment Development

Matching commitment level to confidence level helps ensure clients don't overcommit and set themselves up for failure.

Confidence-focused commitment work:

77. "How confident are you that you could [specific behavior]? What would you be more confident about?"
78. "What commitment would match your current confidence level?"
79. "You're not completely confident about [big change]. What smaller commitment would you feel confident about?"

80. "What would you bet money you could accomplish this week?"
81. "If you had to guarantee success, what would you commit to?"

Commitment Planning

Once someone expresses willingness to make a commitment, helping them create a specific plan increases the likelihood of follow-through.

Planning questions:

82. "When will you do this?"
83. "Where will you be when you make this change?"
84. "What will you do first, second, third?"
85. "Who else needs to know about this commitment?"
86. "What will success look like?"
87. "How will you know if your plan is working?"

Implementation details:

88. "What time of day works best for this commitment?"
89. "What do you need to have in place before you start?"
90. "What might interfere with your plan, and how will you handle it?"
91. "Who or what will support you in keeping this commitment?"
92. "What will remind you to follow through?"

Commitment Maintenance

Helping clients think through how they'll maintain their commitment over time prevents early abandonment when motivation wanes.

Maintenance planning:

93. "What will keep you motivated when the initial excitement wears off?"
94. "How will you recommit when you don't feel like following through?"
95. "What will you tell yourself when this gets difficult?"
96. "Who will you turn to for support when you're struggling?"
97. "How will you celebrate progress along the way?"
98. "What will you do if you have a setback?"

When motivation might fluctuate:

99. "Your motivation is high right now. What will you rely on when motivation is low?"
100. "What would your future self want current self to commit to?"
101. "How will you reconnect with your reasons for change when you forget why you started?"
102. "What commitment would survive your worst mood or most difficult day?"

Multiple Commitment Options

Sometimes clients benefit from having several commitment options to choose from rather than feeling locked into one specific change.

Offering choice in commitment:

103. "You could commit to [option A], [option B], or [option C]. Which appeals to you most?"
104. "What feels more doable—changing [behavior] or changing [different behavior]?"
105. "Would you rather commit to doing something new or stopping something old?"
106. "Which commitment would be harder to break—[option 1] or [option 2]?"
107. "You could start with [small step] or jump into [bigger step]. What fits for you?"

When Clients Won't Commit

Sometimes clients aren't ready to make any specific commitments. This needs to be accepted rather than pushed against.

Responses to commitment avoidance:

108.   "It sounds like you're not ready to commit to specific changes yet."
109.   "Maybe the commitment you're willing to make is to keep thinking about this."
110.   "What if your only commitment was to stay open to the possibility of change?"
111.   "Perhaps you're committing to not making any commitments right now, and that's okay."
112.   "What would need to change for you to feel ready to make a commitment?"

When timing isn't right:

113.   "This might not be the right time for big commitments."
114.   "What would make the timing feel better for making changes?"
115.   "Maybe your commitment is to figure out when you'll be ready to commit."
116.   "What if you committed to having another conversation about this in [timeframe]?"

The Power of Public Commitment

Research shows that commitments made in front of others are more likely to be kept than private commitments.

Exploring public commitment:

117.   "Who would you want to tell about this commitment?"

118.   "What would it be like to share your plan with [important person]?"
119.   "Would it help to have someone check in with you about your progress?"
120.   "How do you feel about making this commitment public versus keeping it private?"
121.   "Who would be most supportive of your commitment to change?"

The Art of Commitment Timing

Knowing when to ask for commitment is crucial. Too early and you might get superficial agreement without real buy-in. Too late and the motivation might have passed. The sweet spot is usually when:

- The client has expressed strong change talk
- They've explored their motivations thoroughly
- They've begun to see themselves as capable of change
- They're asking practical questions about how to change
- They seem emotionally ready to take action

Watch for these signs and trust your instincts about timing. When in doubt, you can ask: "Are you ready to talk about what you might want to do about this, or do you need more time to think?"

Beyond the First Commitment

The goal isn't just to get one commitment but to help clients develop the skill of making and keeping commitments to themselves. This builds self-efficacy and creates momentum for larger changes.

Start with small, achievable commitments that build confidence. Success breeds success, and clients who experience the satisfaction of keeping commitments to themselves become more willing to make bigger commitments later.

The relationship between commitment and change is complex. Commitment without adequate preparation often fails. Preparation without commitment leads nowhere. The art is helping clients find the sweet spot where they're both ready and willing to take action toward positive change.

The Complete MI Practitioner

You now have a complete library of MI phrases and responses for every situation you're likely to encounter. From those crucial first words in opening sessions to the advanced techniques that help people move from thinking about change to actually changing, these scripts provide the language foundation for transformational conversations.

But scripts are just the beginning. The real artistry of MI comes from understanding when to use which response, how to adapt these phrases to your personal style, and how to read the subtle cues that tell you whether you're helping or hindering the change process.

The 500+ phrases in this book aren't meant to be memorized and recited. They're meant to be internalized and adapted, to become part of your natural conversational repertoire. The best MI practitioners sound spontaneous and authentic even while using these proven response patterns.

Take these scripts and make them your own. Practice them until they feel natural. Adapt them to your personality and your clients' needs. Most importantly, use them in service of something larger than technique—the profound human capacity for growth, healing, and positive change.

When you master this language, you don't just become a better counselor. You become someone who helps people discover their own wisdom, strength, and motivation for creating the life they truly want to live.

References

Brehm, S. S., & Brehm, J. W. (2013). *Psychological reactance: A theory of freedom and control*. Academic Press.

Elliot, A. J. (2008). *Handbook of approach and avoidance motivation*. Psychology Press.

Elliott, R., Bohart, A. C., Watson, J. C., & Greenberg, L. S. (2011). Empathy. *Psychotherapy, 48*(1), 43-49.

Hill, C. E., & Knox, S. (2009). Processing the therapeutic relationship. *Psychotherapy Research, 19*(1), 13-29.

Jacobson, N. S., & Addis, M. E. (1993). Research on couples and couple therapy: What do we know? Where are we going? *Journal of Consulting and Clinical Psychology, 61*(1), 85-93.

Janis, I. L., & Mann, L. (1977). *Decision making: A psychological analysis of conflict, choice, and commitment*. Free Press.

Kazdin, A. E. (2007). Mediators and mechanisms of change in psychotherapy research. *Annual Review of Clinical Psychology, 3*, 1-27.

Lambert, M. J., & Barley, D. E. (2001). Research summary on the therapeutic relationship and psychotherapy outcome. *Psychotherapy: Theory, Research, Practice, Training, 38*(4), 357-361.

Miller, W. R., & Rollnick, S. (2013). *Motivational interviewing: Helping people change* (3rd ed.). Guilford Press.

Prochaska, J. O., & DiClemente, C. C. (1983). Stages and processes of self-change of smoking: Toward an integrative model of change. *Journal of Consulting and Clinical Psychology, 51*(3), 390-395.

Prochaska, J. O., & Norcross, J. C. (2018). *Systems of psychotherapy: A transtheoretical analysis* (8th ed.). Cengage Learning.

Rokeach, M. (1973). *The nature of human values.* Free Press.

Rollnick, S., Miller, W. R., & Butler, C. C. (2008). *Motivational interviewing in health care: Helping patients change behavior.* Guilford Press.

Safran, J. D., & Kraus, S. (2014). Alliance ruptures, impasses, and enactments: A relational perspective. *Psychotherapy, 51*(3), 381-387.

Seligman, M. E. P. (1972). Learned helplessness: Annual review of medicine. *Annual Review of Medicine, 23*, 407-412.

Snyder, C. R., Michael, S. T., & Cheavens, J. S. (2000). Hope as a foundation for helping. In C. R. Snyder (Ed.), *Handbook of hope: Theory, measures, and applications* (pp. 3-25). Academic Press.

www.ingramcontent.com/pod-product-compliance
Lightning Source LLC
Chambersburg PA
CBHW072145270326
41931CB00010B/1891